FOUR GLORIOUS YEARS

Mona E Stanton

FOUR GLORIOUS YEARS

Mona E Stanton

Pen Press
London

© Mona Stanton 1996

First Published in Great Britain in 1996 by
Pen Press
Church House
Portland Avenue
London N16 6HJ

ISBN 1 900796 05 8

A catalogue record of this book is available
from the British Library.

Front cover design and illustrations by
Catrina Sherlock, Waves Graphic Design

Printed by Hobbs the Printers Ltd, Totton, Hampshire SO40 3YS

Foreword

With the 50th Anniversary of the end of the Second World War, we've recently been reminded of the Allies' many strategic achievements.

History though, is not just the account of nations' doings, it is also the story of individuals — the personal tales and experiences of people like Mona Stanton. It is also the story of women's lives and their contributions to the war effort.

Allied front lines could only advance if each effort was supported by full mobilisation at home: as well as D-Day, there were all the other days of the war; as well as the battles in France, Africa and the Pacific, there were agonising struggles in hospital wards.

Nearly everyone was called up, in one manner or another, for one special duty or another. For year after year, normal life ceased.

This is a book about one woman's life in wartime; a chronicle that gives a personal dimension to events that might otherwise seem far removed from the world we now know. It is history with a human face.

Catherine Tizard

Dame Catherine Tizard GCMG, DBE
Governor-General of New Zealand

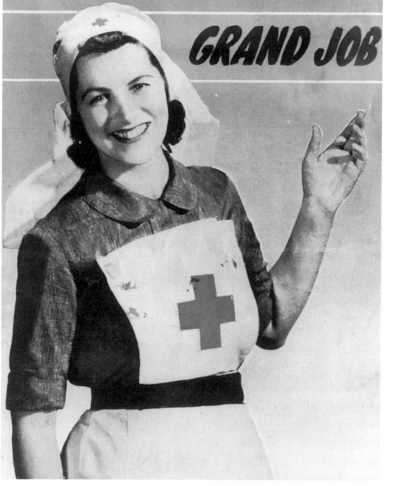

I DECIDE TO JOIN UP

Ever to become a nurse was the last occupation that crossed my mind. I was trained as a shorthand-typist, teleprinting operator, and a telephonist. At the time I was working for the B.B.C. at Evesham, where I had a chance to study the language I wanted too, by conversing with a fellow colleague who broadcast to his own country regularly.

My one ambition was to find a way to rejoin my family who were back in New Zealand. At that time there seemed no hope of my ever being able to do such a thing, as being of conscription age, I was not permitted to leave the country, as all man-power in that country was urgently needed to help in their all out effort to regain peace.

With the ever increasing number of casualties, many of whom would be incapacitated for the rest of their lives, and to see so many friends and colleagues suffer that awful blow: grief; that to help in a more active way was manifesting itself deeper and deeper in my plan to work my way back home. I pondered for some time wondering whether I could possibly be of any more assistance as a nurse, and hoped for an opportunity to serve on a hospital-ship, to give me an opportunity to see my family from time to time.

The attractive posters that were displayed; COME AND JOIN ME IN A GRAND JOB: and WE NEED YOUR HELP: coupled with the constant and persistent call for young women to join the Red Cross, to help to relieve the acute shortages of nurses, I am sure encouraged many to do the same as I did.

For most, they would be able to see their families once a year when they had their annual leaves, but for me, I would probably have to wait till the end of the war.

I had some qualms in changing over from my comparative free and interesting life, and temporarily abandoning my ambition, to the more disciplined life of a nurse. My rather disillusioned impression of a Matron who ruled with a rod of iron, and Sisters that shouted at nurses all day long, was no encouragement. One fact I had to face, was that my family was now safe and sound in New Zealand, and it was up to me to find a way to rejoin them.

I need not have worried about my decision, as in the years that followed, I rather ruefully regretted that I had not taken my full training.

From Evesham I applied to the Red Cross headquarters in London, offering my services as a V.A.D. and was duly accepted after I had passed the necessary medical. I was fortunate in having some very good friends in Tottenham, where I knew I was welcome to stay while I took a series of lectures in First-Aid and Home-Nursing, and then to do the necessary sixty hours on a hospital ward.

The class was not very big, but was made up of girls from all walks of life, who were keenly interested and preferred to become nurses for their war-time occupation, in preference to being man-powered into one of the vital war-industries, which was so equally essential for Britain's survival.

None of us expected to pass the elementary exam at the end of the fortnight. Our biggest problem was how to remember all the bones of the body, and where they all belonged. There just seemed to be so many, that we couldn't see how anyone could remember them all, or put them in the right places. As for pressure points, I was sure that I would tell the examiner that the occipital was at the back of the knee. Bandaging was always a problem, as it always used to slip from one's hand, and roll across the floor. It did too at the exam, and cost me five points, but we all managed to pass with reasonably good marks. Next came the hospital training. We were posted to different hospitals, and I never saw my class mates again.

Since I was staying in Tottenham, I began my training at the Middlesex County Hospital, in October 1942. The Battle of Britain was over and heroically won, but there was no sign yet of how long the war would continue, or tragically how many more decent young lives would be sacrificed. War was as much a woman's job as a man's, and the wanton destruction of young and innocent children, the aged, as well as those in hospital all needed care, and I resolved to do all I could to adapt myself to my new way of life.

I presented myself at nine in the morning to the Matron, and was assigned to the Alexandra ward. On arrival, feeling very lost indeed, I was given a long white gown and what I took to be a serviette. Nurses were buzzing round in all directions carrying trays, dusters, and vases of flowers, in and out of a very long, but very severely tidy ward. The first thing I felt I had to learn, was how to walk very quickly indeed, and look efficient even if I wasn't.

As I donned my new mode of dress, I found to my horror, that it reached tight to my ankles. I spent some time looking and asking for, and eventually getting sufficient safety-pins to put a sizable hem on it. As for the serviette, I was at a loss to know why I had been given such a thing. Feeling more lost

3

than ever I found a very stern looking person behind a very large desk, which was covered in papers, and asked what it was for. With sarcasm she informed me it was my cap. This made things even worse. I asked the first nurse I saw how on earth I could make a cap out of it. Showing kindness and understanding to a now very bewildered greenhorn, I duly had a cap on, and was told the person behind the desk was the ward-sister, whose bark was worse than her bite, and I'd soon get used to it.

My first job was to help to make the beds. This seemed unnecessary as they were all tidy, but we made them just the same. Most of the patients had a pleasant word as we made their beds, while others seemed to be in another world. Some were paler than I had ever seen anyone before. As we got to the end of the ward it seemed very strange to see an elderly patient, whose leg was raised high in the air, encased in plaster and supported on a sling. I was to learn that she had tripped on the pavement and had a fractured femur. Further down on the other side of the ward I felt very sad to see a tiny little girl with her head swathed in bandages, and her expressionless face almost as white as the sheets around her. She was the pet of the ward, and I felt so happy when I had finished my fortnight on the ward that she was improving so much she could smile again.

Next came a very speedy walk down miles of corridors for morning tea, to be hurriedly swallowed in a very noisy cafeteria, milling with nurses, who always seemed to be laughing, and to have so much to talk about. The constant noisy rattle of cutlery and crockery, was strong competition for the endless babble of cheerful voices, broken intermittently by a bright infectious laugh which seems to be the hall-mark whenever nurses gathered. No sooner had we arrived when it was time to return to the ward again down the same long corridors, at the same breakneck speed.

On returning I landed the job of what was called dirty-nurse. Given no time to ponder over this title, I found I had to precede the senior nurse and to move the screens from one patient to the next. Although having nothing to do with the actual handling of a dressing, I too, had to wear a mask. At first this was very uncomfortable and seemed to impede one's breathing, and made you feel very hot and moist and stuffy around the mouth and nose. It was always a relief to be able to slip it down for a breather while transferring the screens from one bed to the next. I found this part of nursing very interesting, and became quite absorbed in what I was doing.

As we passed from bed to bed, she gave me a quiet and brief explanation of each patient's ailment, and the necessary treatment. This proved more and more interesting. When we came to a very pale patient that I had noticed while making the beds, I glanced at the nurse, and became aware of a great feeling of devotion she seemed to transmit. With great care, she had to do a dressing for the patient's recent kidney operation. I had never witnessed such tenderness before, as the patient was so ill she had to be handled with great patience and skill. Never before had I seen such an enormous wound. After completing the outsize dressing, I was asked if I felt ill. It hadn't affected me in any way, as I had become so engrossed in the whole work of art, I was rather surprised at her question. She was rather surprised when I simply said "No", and remarked it was very seldom such dressings didn't affect a new nurse. She suggested that I took up nursing as a career. I was interested in the work I was doing for the first time, and bucked by her remark that I almost considered it, but didn't want to jeopardise any chance I might have in the future of getting on a hospital-ship. So I let it slide, and anyhow I was too scared in case a patient died. Then with horror I was stung into realisation that no patient on any ward I work on must ever die. Now lost in a world of my own, together we went on to do many and varied dressings, from a stitched and septic finger, to complete hysterectomies. As we approached the wee girl I was told that Sister had to help with that one. When we had completed all the other dressings, I had to let Sister know that the nurse was ready to do the mastoid dressing. As they skillfully and carefully cleaned and redressed the wound the little girl's screams were something I had never heard before, and they were to haunt me for many months. It bothered me so much I began to wonder if I could be any use as a nurse after all, and at my first opportunity asked the nurse why she screamed so much. With a kind and gentle smile, she explained that the dressing had to be done, and that the patient was in no danger now. I would have to get used to such things as time went on. Still feeling disconsolate, I was relieved to see the child settled down once more. I remember how much I admired the selfless devotion a real nurse showed towards her patients.

From dressings I had to take round cups of tea which had arrived from the kitchens. Some of the patients seemed to be more friendly by this time and I found them very cheerful. Panning time soon arrived and even this held no displeasure for me. Following this I had to help to tidy the ward again and straighten up the beds. Curiously this was a great relaxation after the work I had been doing.

It seemed so peaceful and quiet and slowly I walked up the ward, pondering over my new type of work with a sense of duty and a feeling of satisfaction at really helping those who could not altogether help themselves. As I was dreaming I heard a voice saying "Nurse!", and again "Nurse!", but continued to dream lost in thought. The tranquillity was broken by a sudden "Answer when you are spoken to!".

I snapped into consciousness. "Oh that's me," I faltered through my daydreaming. How strange it seemed to be called

Nurse after so short a time on a ward. What a raucous voice Sister seemed to have too. In front of all the patients she sharply remarked, "You must go and see immediately what the patient wants when they call you Nurse. It may be urgent."

Somehow, although feeling humiliated and annoyed, I could only answer, "Yes Sister," and went to see what was wanted.

Apologising for having caused me to be spoken to like that, she went on to say that she hadn't realised I had only been on the ward for a few hours, and began chatting. As my uniform was different from the others, she was interested to know why. When I told her that I was only doing my sixty hours to become a V.A.D.(Voluntary Aid Detachment) and hoped to get into the Navy, she was even more interested, and gave me her son's address. As he was about my own age she asked me to look him up if I was sent to Chatham. I felt very shy at this request, and told her that if I had to put up with being spoken to like I was a moment ago, I would never get that far.

"Oh you mustn't worry, she speaks like that to all the nurses, but she doesn't mean any harm. You watch her when she changes the little girl's dressings, and you'll see how wonderful she really is."

So the next time she changed the dressing, I did watch her. I had never before seen a battle-axe be so kind and gentle, and show such tenderness. I changed my opinion instantly, but changed it back just as instantly when she saw me doing nothing, and once again her voice battered against my eardrums with, "Don't stand there doing nothing!. If you've got nothing to do, take all the flowers out, wash the vases and change the water, and put them back again, and let me know when you have finished!"

"Yes Sister" I again replied meekly, as somehow one's antagonism seems to automatically be suppressed by the natural respect for decisive and conclusive orders, given by those whom one has a subconcious trust and confidence in.

Oh dear what an existence, but with pleasure I spent about an hour walking peacefully backward and forwards, taking each vase from each locker, washing it, changing the water, and replacing it again. When I had finished I reported as requested and was sharply told to go to lunch.

As the senior nurse was to go too, again we had another speedy walk, down miles of corridors, to the cafeteria, but this time I was able to keep up the pace a little better. After we returned from lunch, I was very relieved to find Sister was off duty. The senior nurse was in charge, and asked me if I had ever taken temperatures. I told her I had learned how to do it at our lectures. She asked me to take them but to record them on paper, so she could check them and show me how to enter them on the temperature charts. After the first few, she was satisfied I could take them correctly, as well as the pulse and respirations. I loved this part of my work, and soon found I was to do them daily, I also found it was no trouble to mark the charts correctly. I was very fascinated at the varying degrees in temperatures of each patient. The rest of the day was very peaceful, but never before had I felt so tired as when I was on the tram going back to Tottenham.

On arrival at my friend's place, it was heaven to flop in an easy-chair, and at last, I could dispense with my pins and take up the large hem on my uniform in a more orthodox manner. Feeling very tired after what seemed to be a very hard day's work, as up till then, I had always had to sit down to work, but now I had to run round. I didn't waste any time getting to bed after tea. As sleep began to relax my mind and tired body, I could hear again our wee girl's screams. It bothered me and I wondered should I really carry on. Pondering a good deal over this, I satisfied my mind by realizing I could not accommodate myself all in one day, and firmly resolved to at least finish my fortnight of actual hospital duty, as I was finding satisfaction in my new occupation and environment.

The following day after I had taken the temperatures in the early afternoon, I had to assist in giving my first blanket-bath. After surrounding the patient with screens, and removing each piece of bed linen, folding them neatly on to a chair, and leaving one blanket to cover the patient, we carefully and systematically washed each patient thoroughly. Mostly we were able to do this alone, but with the very ill patients, an extra nurse was sometimes needed, in order to lessen any strain on the patient. Tenderness, care and thoroughness was very important, if the patient had been in bed for any length of time. It was a mark of bad nursing to allow any patient to become a victim of bed-sores. At first it seemed to be rather futile just to rub the pressure points, with a thin covering of soap till it disappeared, and then giving a good firm rub with methylated spirits, and dusting the area over with powder. Many years later, I was to see a very large bed-sore, caused by the lack of this treatment, and realised how necessary it was.

Blanket-bathing time always seemed to be a peaceful and chatty time, and it was then I came to know more about my patients. It must have been a welcome change for them too, to have a quiet chat within the privacy of the screens. Life seemed very quiet and peaceful, as the senior nurse arrived on duty that day, and came to ask if she could assist in any way. I was managing quite well, but she gave a hand, as I had so many baths to do, and when we had finished, I asked her, if she had done any other kind of work before taking up nursing. Looking into her serene deep blue eyes, that I had noticed while we were doing dressings, she replied "No, I had always wanted to be a nurse and wouldn't change my life for anything." How much I admired a real nurse.

On arrival next moring, I slipped passed Sister's office, I heard her voice as I approached my ward, and felt almost at home as I fitted in to the routine of another day's work. I glanced first at our wee girl, and she seemed much the same.

9

We had a new patient, whose face was covered in enormous burn blisters.

Early in the afternoon a message came through to say that we had to prepare for a patient with a fractured spine. As I was the only available nurse at the time, Sister asked me to prepare a fracture-bed. Quickly casting my mind back to my lectures, I hoped I could remember how to make it. How I wished there was someone else to help me, and to show me where the necessary things were, and to check it to see if I had made it up correctly when I had finished. Working and thinking over and over again of what I should get, I found and placed the boards on the bed-wire, and realising how hard it would be for the patient, I made up the bed. Sister came to check the bed, as I waited for a blast, but none came. She only complimented me on my work, and I felt I was in her good books at last. After we had received the patient, taken her temperature, and made her as comfortable as we could, with relief another nurse returned from lunch. Walking back down the ward, feeling Sister wasn't so bad after all, a patient summoned me, and asked my why I didn't take up nursing seriously. "I think you would make a good nurse," she ventured.

With a chuckle I said "No fear, I've got other ideas and I only hope I don't strike too many battle-axes, although she's not bad at times."

"No Nurse!" struck from behind. "Go into the sluice-room and sterilize all the bed-pans!" Smiling to my patient I disappeared to the sluice-room for as long as I could stay there, to keep out of trouble, and hoping she would soon go off duty so that I could emerge from my oversized turkish-bath.

Long before I was anywhere near finished my solitary task, Sister asked me to take all the temperatures, as our only other nurse was too busy to take them. Although I should have been back at my friend's place, I then had to give various medicines and tablets to the patients who required them. Without realizing the time I carried on to treat all pressure points where required, and finally help those who couldn't help themselves, to be comfortable and settled for the night. Just as I was told I could leave another patient was admitted suffering from an abdominal cancer. Her outlook was very grim, but I was pleased to see her settled and comfortable before I left the ward. Three new patients in an already overcrowded ward with an acute shortage of staff, was sufficient to dispel any begrudgery of the extra hours one put on the wards, and to lessen any temptation I had to give it up, and to strengthen my determination to carry on.

It was a big surprise to learn our most recent patient had died during the night, when I began my duties the next morning. How thankful I felt I wasn't there.

The rest of the fortnight went off very quickly and peacefully it seemed to me, with patients being admitted and discharged in a continuous round. Our dear little girl remained with us, but with colour returning to her cheeks, and the nurses spending a little more time once each day playing with her, for very short periods. Her screams were no longer to be heard, instead her happy laughter, seemed to cheer the whole ward, and she too was soon for discharge. With one more day to go, I found I had learned how to take and record temperatures, pulses, and respirations accurately, blanket-bath single handed, except for very ill patients, give medicines, do minor dressings, and keep out of Sister's way.

Now feeling that I could be more of a help than a hindrance, and that I could go on, I had to help Sister receive a patient who had been involved in a street accident. What a mess. This was the worst case I had seen, and was rather overawed at the thought, of seeing such cases in the future. Sister sent me to get a nightdress. Hoping to remain in peace, I climbed to the top of the linen cupboard, and found a white one which was far nicer than the ones we had been using. Handing it to Sister it immediately landed in my face with a loud "Take that back!". Bewildered by this sudden outburst, I returned to the linen cupboard, and sat on the clothes basket nursing my lovely nighty, ignoring another nurse who was sorting linen and methodically putting it away.

Following a few minutes silence, she asked me what I was doing. "I thought you were working with Sister?"

Slowly and thoughtfully I replied, "I was, but when I gave her the nighty she asked for, she threw it at me and told me to take it back. I'm jolly glad I finish tomorrow, I'll never get used to her. I hope all Sisters aren't the same." Without warning my colleague burst out laughing. Now feeling indignant I said "You can keep your nursing. I can't see what's funny in that."

"You poor thing," she replied, "you gave her a shroud."

"Oh no!" I exclaimed, and then I too, could see the funny side of it.

Such was life on a hospital ward. Tragedy, interest, hard work, devotion, thoughtfulness, relief, respect, gentleness, understanding, and most of all, a sense of humour to carry you on and on, where your own personal tiredness ceases even to be felt.

My last day on the ward seemed almost sad when Sister handed me her report on my fortnight's work on the ward. I had to take the sealed envelope to Matron. I knew that I had been in hot-water too often to command a favourable one, and walked thoughtfully to her office, wondering what I would do if I was not accepted as a nurse.

Gingerly knocking on Matron's door, she immediately asked me to come in. Responding to her "Good-morning," I handed her my envelope.

Silently reading the report she quietly said, "Sister is interested to know if you would consider taking your training, as she would like to have you on her ward."

Stunned into blank amazement by her request, and incapable of comprehending at that moment, I said "But she can't, I was always in trouble."

"No nurse, she likes a girl with spirit, you just don't understand her, I always send as many of my recruits as I can to her ward, as she is an excellent but strict, and a very fair Sister. She has given you an excellent report. I would like you to consider it."

Remembering the two-fold purpose I had in mind, I could only answer, "Thank you Matron, but I want to join the Navy to get on to a hospital-ship, in the hope that I can get home from time to time, but I am very pleased to know I can now be accepted as a V.A.D. in the Red Cross."

"Alright nurse," she replied, "but if you ever do decide to take up nursing, we would be very happy to have you here, I am very pleased with your report."

Leaving Matron's office I meditated for a few minutes on our favourable conversation, but went immediately and phoned Red Cross Headquarters, to tell them of my success, and was advised to return to my civil occupation, until I was called up.

Optimistically ringing my previous supervisor, who was at Broadcasting House, I explained my position to her and was fortunate as she had a vacancy on the teleprinters in London. So I was able to return to the B.B.C. to await my call-up.

In order to determine whether I could serve in the Royal Navy or would have to go to one of the other services, I called in at Headquarters. I was told I would have to go where I was needed most, so stipulated that I only wanted to go into the Navy, but held back my secret wish to serve on a hospital-ship in order that I may have a chance of visiting my family from time to time.

For the next two months, I thoroughly enjoyed my work in the news-room of Broadcasting House, but hoping each day that I would get into the Navy. A fortnight before Xmas I received my call-up, and to my great joy and relief had been posted to the Royal Naval Hospital Haslar.

Handing in my resignation at the B.B.C. I spent the next fortnight purchasing as much of my uniform as I could with the very limited amount of money I had.

The greatest gift anyone can have when you are in an overseas country, is friends. I seemed to have more than my fair share, of really sincere ones, and knew I would never be at a loss of where to go on leaves, as their doors were permanently open to me at any time.

On receiving my travel-warrant to Gosport, a great feeling of pride and excitement filled my heart as I was really on the first leg of my ambition. Calling into the news-room to say good-bye to my friends as promised before leaving for Haslar, it gave me a very comforting feeling to be asked to call in and see them if I ever came to London again, so I kept my B.B.C. pass. I felt a little sad too, looking from the train window as I waved good-bye to Phyl and Eva. I had such a wonderful time staying with them since my return to London to take my lectures, and do my hospital training, and then the two months back at Broadcasting House.

As the train slowly pulled away and gained speed, the monotonous rhythmic clacking of the train wheels on the lines lulled me into a dozy and thoughtful state, and my mixed feelings of excitement and sadness gave way to deep thought. At last I was a Mobile V.A.D. and in the Navy. Oblivious of my fellow passengers, I wondered how long it would be, before I could try for a hospital-ship. Would I meet any more girls from New Zealand? What would life in the Navy be like? Were the Sisters very strict? Would I have to nurse really badly

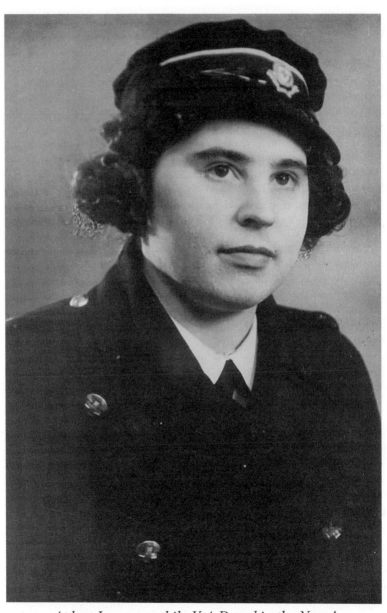

At last I was a mobile V.A.D and in the Navy!

injured patients? How long would it be now before I could get home, and most important of all, would I be be able to stand up to whatever was asked of me? The train sped on and on, but I could see nothing from the window, as it was such horrible weather.

The train arrived at Portsmouth late on a very damp and foggy afternoon. A naval Petty-Officer was on the look-out for me, and for two other girls that had travelled on the same train. Together with our luggage, we were taken to the liberty boat. The biting cold salty spray smacked and stung our faces, as the boat bounced up and down ploughing her way through the fog to Gosport. On arrival we were met by another naval escort, and transferred to a naval van, and taken on to the nurse's quarters at the hospital.

HASLAR

A senior V.A.D. greeted us at the door and took us immediately for a very welcome cup of tea, before we were to report to the Commandant's office, we were shown the notice-board which was to be the silent voice of all our future movements; of the wards we would be sent on, the times of our duties, the times of the various church services, and any other information that was relevent to each one of us. The mail-board too, an everlasting companion from where we would daily hope to receive mail from our friends and families, both near and far.

Arriving at our yet unknown commandant's office, while waiting in turn to be interviewed I could only feel I was now a member of Royal Naval personnel, and from now on civilian dress was a thing of the past, as uniform had to be worn at all times. There seemed a whole interesting life ahead of me. The calm efficiency and happy atmosphere I had come in contact with so far, gave one a sense of companionship and encouragement. I was eager to really get started.

When my turn came to be interviewed a deliberate clear "Come in!" sounded through the closed door, in answer to my gentle knock.

"Good afternoon, Nurse. Sit down please," she requested as I walked in, and continued to neatly place papers in a folder with the particulars of the nurse she had seen previously to me, but quietly chatting about my journey, and how happy all the nurses were, putting me completely at ease. Automatically placing some fresh forms in front of her, she asked for my name, date of birth, next of kin, home adresss, any illnesses and so on. Filling in each detail as I gave them to her.

"You're a long way from home," she enquiringly remarked.

"Yes I know. Are there any other New Zealand girls here?" I enquired.

"No, I haven't had one so far, but if I do, I will let you know. Tomorrow you will have another medical and be shown round the hospital, and you will have a day to settle in. The ward you will be sent to will be on the notice-board. All V.A.D.s have to be in their dormitories by nine o'clock and lights out at ten-thirty, unless you have a late pass. You are permitted one a week till midnight. Sleeping out passes are granted to those who have friends or relations in Portsmouth. I think you will be very happy here but if you have any worries or need advice, don't hesitate to come to me and I will do all I can to help and advise you. I have a lot of time for New Zealanders."

This comforting remark made me feel very welcome and proud.

Handing me yet another form to fill in, one to be returned to her office and one copy for myself, I was asked to get another V.A.D. to witness it. More forms, more medicals, and I wondered if this procedure was repeated when you went on draft. Leaving Madam Waistell's office I was extremely impressed with her deliberate but kindly manner. Now left with the nurse who had taken charge of us, we were shown to a very long dormitory, partitioned with a doorless doorway.

Along each side of the dormitory were double bunks separated by individual lockers. Wardrobes were shared with about half a dozen of us. There were sixty of us in the dorm. Some of the nurses I understood had only been at Haslar for a couple of weeks, and some had been there for months. Being a Base hospital, one never knew how long it would be before you were drafted to another hospital or where. After unpacking our belongings and washing and freshening up, we were taken to the mess and issued with an enamel plate, one knife, one fork, one spoon and a cup that was so thick and heavy that I am sure not even a bomb could crack it. Once again there were nurses everywhere. Only this time they looked very impressive with the scarlet red cross emblazoned on the bib of their aprons covering a pale blue indoor military style frock and wearing what we called the feather duster cap, centred also with a small crimson red cross.

In amongst the red cross nurses were a few in St. John's uniform distinguished by the St. John's insignia embroidered on the bib of their aprons and on the front of their caps. Many St. John's nurses joined the Red Cross and came under the jurisdiction of the service in which they had volunteered and had been sent.

The evening meal was in progress and we had to line up to be served from an enormous heated steel dinner trolley. Any of the first course that was left had to be scraped off your plate into a bin for that purpose, and the sweets were then served on the same plate. Each V.A.D. had to wash her own cutlery and crockery and be responsible for it. It was fun to be militarized and taking an active part in the hub of a war-time occupation.

Gathering in the sitting room after tea, although the atmosphere was friendly, conversation was rather reserved,owing to the short length of time most of us had been there. After filling in my form and getting it witnessed, I made

19

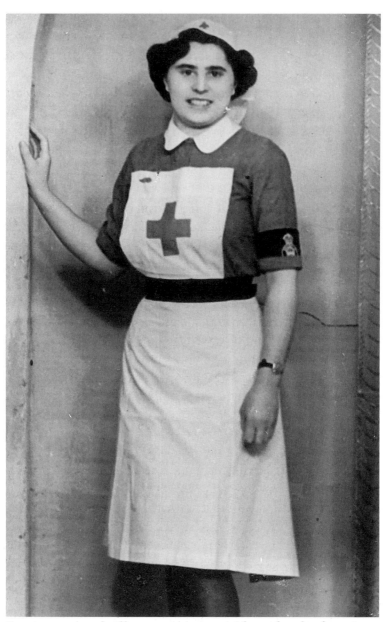

It was a great thrill to get into my uniform for the first time.

my way to the dorm and was thankful to climb into my upper bunk and relax with a book. Sharp at 9 p.m., Madam came through the dorm to see that all nurses were in, except those who had late passes, and lights *were* out at 10.30 p.m.

The following morning it was a great thrill to get into my indoor uniform for the first time. Lining up behind a very well made up blonde, I wistfully smiled to myself as Madam who was serving breakfast queried, "Did you cut your mouth on a jam tin?"

"No Madam."

"Well take that red stuff off your mouth before you go on duty. You're a nurse," she reminded her. "Get that hair off your collar" she told another. Militarized I thought, but we do have a job to do.

After breakfast a handful of us were taken for our medicals. I wanted to giggle when the doctor asked if any of us had flat feet. Passed as medically fit we were then shown around the hospital. As we passed the operating theatre, the smell of ether seemed to permeate every corridor. We were taken to the small serene chapel snuggled as near to the centre of the vast hospital as it could be, and was used by all denominations at varying times.

Beneath the great concrete piles of this massive hospital I was very impressed with the miniature theatre, that had been built in order to afford the maximum protection from a bombing raid. Here many an emergency operation had been carried out on casualties suffered from an attack.

Rows and rows of triple tiered bunks filled the basements. All patients were transferred from the upper wards every night, as bombing attacks were often made. Patients who were unable to be moved, had to take their chance, but there was always a nurse who preferred to remain on duty and take her chance too. This duty was purely voluntary, and as far as I know every nurse volunteered for it.

Smoking of course was prohibited on duty, but during a raid it was permissable. To be standing alongside a completely helpless patient, with the ominous thud of falling bombs, making everything tremble, gave one dutch courage. To hear the very familiar whine, followed by a close thud, brought only "gee that was close, too bad he missed, let's have another cigarette." The bravery of the nurses under bombardment was to be greatly admired. Many casualties had been suffered amongst them as a result of their shining example.

Petitioned off at various intervals from the main line of bunks, were enclosures, where every night eight nurses slept, fully clothed, in order to assist should an emergency arise.

After spending a most interesting morning being shown around the hospital, war-time conditions seemed ironically exciting.

Crossing the large forecourt that separated the nurse's quarters from the main hospital, I wondered how I would ever find my way around. Going automatically to the notice-board, I learned I had to report to Ward B 1 the following morning.

At lunch I was befriended by another nurse who was feeling almost as lost as me. As we had a whole afternoon to ourselves, together we went to Portsmouth and looked around. It seemed so peaceful, and quiet, that it was hard to believe there was a war in progress. The severe bomb damage bore witness that it was no illusion. Nelson's ship permanently anchored in Portsmouth harbour was significant of Britain's heroism and traditional Naval supremacy.

Returning for tea we were joined by more nurses, and invited along to Toc H in the evening.

"What do you do there?" I enquired.

"It's a club and you can get a cup of tea and a cake or a bun. Sometimes there's a lot of New Zealanders there, you may meet someone you know" was suggested to me.

By the time we left to go ashore to Toc H, there were about half a dozen of us, and it was fascinating to hear the wide variety of English accents. So I was no oddity except for land distance.

"Make way for the nurses!" heralded us as we ventured inside. The club was so packed that it was almost impossible to find a seat among the sardined sailors, shrouded in cigarette smoke.

"Ow long ya bin ere?" we were asked.

"Only a few days," came the reply.

"Wat abart comin to the pictures, it's too crarded ere?" we were asked.

"Why not?" we seemed to transmit to one another, and away we went with unknown partners forgetting we had to be in by nine.

As we were returning and neared the hospital we realized we would be a.w.o.l. Chatting happily together I remarked "I hope we don't get caught." One nurse who had been at Haslar for close on a month directed us to a hole in the fence, some distance from the main gate so that we wouldn't be reported at least. It was then up to us not to be seen in the grounds. None of us got caught, and to our relief found Madam had not missed us.

Not wishing to be late on duty the next morning, as I had first to find my ward, I went to breakfast early, and after asking almost everyone I met en route to ward B 1, I eventually got there on time. B 1 was minor surgical. The whole atmosphere was entirely different from the rigidity of a civilian hospital. For one thing most of the patients were young men, whose injuries were either not too severe, or they had recovered sufficiently from severe wounds and were well on the mend. A very cheery good morning came from most of the men, as they were in reasonably merry mood being so near to Christmas.

For a few minutes I saw nothing to do. As I passed an older man's bed, he greeted me with "Well, well, well, what are you doing with a silver fern - met up with Kiwis already?"

"No I haven't seen one, but that is my home," I told him. This remark touched off an avalanche of his exploits to and from the Pacific, as a cook on the P.&O. Liner "Cathay". Before any conversation could take place, "Nurse would you do the arm dressing?" was asked of me.

"Come back when you finish?" my patient asked as I left to do the dressing.

Standing alongside the dressing trolley was a tall patient, wearing a jacket over his white shirt. "Is it your dressing I have to do?" I enquired.

"Yes nurse, you only have to use meths and rub it in well," he told me, as he began removing his jacket sleeve. To my horror his whole arm came off. I was speechless and could only drink in the sickening realization that this rugged young man, would have to go through life with only one arm. The other was artificial. Commandeering my self-control, and suppressing the nauseating feeling that seemed to shock my whole system, I did exactly as I was asked to, and thanked my guardian angel for giving me the strength to overcome my emotional shock. As soon as the task was completed, my shock must have registered visibly, as although not fainting, I became aware of Sister asking me if I was alright. Replying in the affirmative, she asked a nurse who had ushered me to the ward galley to make me a cup of tea.

While I was drinking it, my patient came in to apologize for not having warned me, but to my mind apologies were not necessary, and I had learnt that nothing would make me turn back.

Fully recovered I returned to my older patient, as I was rather interested to hear what he wanted to talk about, as I had sailed as a passenger on the "Cathay". The world is certainly a very small place, as after spending some time sifting and sorting dates, it turned out that he had made the cake for my fourteenth birthday which I spent travelling through the Gulf of Sardinia on my way to England with my family. "I wouldn't mind just one of the eggs I put in that cake right now!" he laughed.

"You ought to be back in New Zealand now," he remarked, and seemed quite concerned when I told him my family had returned but I was too old to leave the country. He laughed heartily. "What made you join the Navy?" he enquired.

"Oh dear it's a long story," I told him. "Before I joined up I applied to try to join the New Zealand nursing service and get on a hospital ship as far back as August 1942, in the hopes of getting home. The New Zealand Intelligence Officer in London, made enquiries to New Zealand, but had been advised that there was no shortage of applicants over there, so therefore they could not accept enlistments from here. So I thought the best thing I could do was to make the best of it here and join up hoping to nurse my way across."

I spent quite a lot of time talking to that patient, when I wasn't busy, as it was a very slender link with home.

When lunch time came, connecting with other nurses on my way back to the quarters, I had the shock of my life to find my bunk unmade. My companions looked surprised too. "Madam couldn't have been round this morning or you would have found it on the deck," said one. How lucky can you be I thought. Getting in late last night, and forgetting to make my bunk this morning. I'm going to make darn sure I don't trip a third time, or I will get caught.

War or no war, Christmas day brought with it a Christmas dinner. The wards were skeleton staffed as much as possible to enable as many nurses as could be spared to have Christmas dinner with their own families. The friendly thought and

25

consideration by sisters, nurses, doctors and patients, left nothing to be desired in cooperation for a very pleasant evening. Madam Waistell endeared herself to us all, with her sincere little speech and good wishes.

When dinner was over, I collected my pillow, and found my way to the basement passing the rows and rows of bunks, till I eventually came to our own sleeping quarters for the night. Two nurses were already there, and the other five soon appeared. One of them gave me the impression she was very restive and seemed to have difficulty in settling down. A feeling of uncertainty crept over me. I was mystified when she began screaming, and became hysterical, and rushed out with her pillow. One of the other nurses followed her, and after a time returned.

"Whatever is the matter?" I had to ask.

"She suffers from claustrophobia, and has tried often to take her turn down here but the same thing happens every time." Hoping there would be no raid we settled down for the night.

"Wakey, wakey!" shouted by an S.B.A. (Sick Berth Attendant) as he walked along the rows of patients brought me to my senses next morning. Running a comb through our hair and hugging our pillows, we made our way back out into daylight dodging the day staff who had already commenced to move the patients back to their wards. The fresh morning air outside, although bitterly cold, was very welcome indeed.

With breakfast over and not feeling the affects of this abnormal way of life, I went on duty again, now more as a matter of course. "I want you to help with the burn case this morning nurse," I was asked when I arrived.

God worked many miracles during the war, and surely our patient who had had more than two thirds of his body burnt, was one of them. He was known to us as the miracle man. Apart from most of his body being scarred by severe burns he had no skin, and very little flesh left on his legs which were kept covered with lassars paste. His cheerful presence in the ward made him a great favourite of us all. Not once did he give any indication of the acute agonizing suffering he'd had to endure.

No sooner had we completed this dressing, and began walking towards the end of the ward, when we were met by an S.B.A, wheeling in another patient concealed by blankets and bandages. "Here's another one for you nurse," was casually implicated. Together we lifted him from the trolley and put him into bed clothes and all. Only his shoes were removed. Our S.B.A. was replaced by Sister, and together we were able to change him from his dirty blood stained clothes, into clean pyjamas and soon had recorded his T.P.R. "Change the dressing please nurse will you," and left me to it.

Momentarily I summed up the job in hand. Having been exposed to the elements for some time, as he was a despatch rider, and had hit an army truck head on, he was very tired and muddy and the bandage covering his entire head was stained with dry blood which had stuck fast to his hair and scalp. Though obviously speedily but deftly applied, it covered an unknown wound, which was yet to be bared to reveal the nature of the injuries he had received.

Carefully soaking each layer of adhered bandage with saline, it gradually yielded to my removing it inch by inch. Applying a clean dressing and fresh capeline, I breathed a sigh of relief at the whole procedure going off without a hitch, but most important of all, no discomforture to my patient. Unaccompanied the doctor arrived soon after to examine him, and passed a very complimentary remark, on whoever had applied the bandage. A feeling of gratification ran through me and I hoped all my work would be as successful, and that it was not just a fluke.

As I was leaving the ward I joined up with one of my colleagues who informed me that she had a New Zealand patient and he would like to meet me as I was from home. Giving me his room number and the time I could pop in and see him, she left me as she was on her way to the dispensary. I looked forward to meeting him at my first opportunity.

It was two days before I had the remotest chance of paying my social call. Expectantly knocking on his door, excited with the prospects of a fair dinkum yarn, he asked me to come in.

"Oh hello, so you are the New Zealand nurse," greeted me as I walked in. What a supercilious type of Kiwi I thought, was I supposed to be wearing a cloak of Kiwi feathers, or a piupiu. "Where are you from?" he enquired.

"Auckland," I replied feeling as flat as a pancake.

"Oh so am I. I went to Mount Albert Grammar," he informed me with great affectation.

"I only got as far as the Mount Albert School, and then we moved to Henderson," I answered him, not enjoying myself at all, and was pleased to leave. If that joker reckons he is a Kiwi, I'm a wallaby I thought as I left his room.

For some unknown reason as soon as my month was up in ward B1, I was not moved. It became as much a part of me as I of it, and I was really enjoying my first few weeks as a Naval nurse.

Orders had come through that as many patients as possible were to be sent home, and we knew that something was afoot. Naturally with less patients in the wards, we occupied ourselves after our routine work had been done in chatting casually to our patients who still required hospital care.

Late one afternoon while doing a knee dressing, the stillness and peaceful contented low mumble of our remaining patients quietly talking to one another was suddenly silenced, by the garrulous and excited unintelligible yelling from the far end of the ward. Instantly struck with alarm and consternation, I looked towards the area of the sudden disturbance and felt bewildered, and not unafraid to witness two very flustered looking S.B.A.s, who, with miraculous skill, were successfully wheeling and keeping a wildly thrashing patient on a moving trolley, returning him to his ward from the operating theatre. I learned from Sister later that this was a rare occurance, and I accepted it as an individual idiosyncrasy to anesthesia. Completing the knee dressing I was doing, "Don't go to New Zealand without me, or I'll be offended!" fell on my ears as I left the ward.

Returning to my quarters that night the notice-board bore the news that I was to go on leave. More proof that something was afoot as with so many less patients we were over-staffed. Proceeding the following day on leave, in as dismal and as foggy weather as I had journeyed down in, it was somewhat of a relief to arrive in London. As we stepped from the carriage a polite voice coming through the loud speakers above the noisy platform, was issuing forth with "Would all V.A.D.s on leave from Haslar please return on the next train!" This was repeated several times, so our leave consisted of a long tiring journey, changing trains, and resigning ourselves to a along journey back. Our spirits were high, and bore no trace of disappointment.

The following morning I was to report back on to ward B1. Boomerang I thought, but what a boomerang. The whole of the nursing staff had been working ceaselessly, as the British had bombed Dieppe, and Portsmouth was getting hell as a reprisal. The half empty wards were over flowing and more casualties expected. Off duty times were mythical. Where a life was in danger there was no room for apathetical complacency, or lack of confidence, and every one was far too busy to think of themselves and thought only of the patients.

Passing quickly down the long corridors I stopped dead in my tracks to the gruesome wailing of the air raid siren. All patients were to go below. Every nurse, sister, and S.B.A., and capable patients pushed those who were immobile in wheelchairs, or on stretchers, and assisted those on crutches to as much safety as the basements could afford. In my ward there was a patient with a fractured spine, and it fell to me to remain with him. Stricken with fear, stabilized only with the knowledge that to move him would mean death for him. I knew my guardian angel would guard us both, we settled down to be mischievous and smoked on duty. Holding our breaths as each death warning whine came closer, we teased one another, as to how well we could count the thuds, and how long the trembling hospital would take to shake to bits or what part was hit. For what seemed ages we remained there, until the all clear was sounded. Gradually the pathetic trail of wounded began to return, and before they had reached the wards again, the raid warning sounded again, and back they all had to go. Sister came to relieve me, but somehow I preferred to remain where I was, and felt my patient's life was as good as my own.

This nightmare went on intermittently for days and nights. Among the ever increasing casualties was a ship's cat. The men had been torpedoed and one of the survivors had been able to save their cat, which was badly injured. It was operated on, given a bed, and a bed ticket. As each man required an operation from that ship was taken to theatre, they were permitted the company of their cat. This unselfish consideration, made me feel every patient I nursed a hero in his own right, and well worth anything I had to be called upon to do.

When the raids lessened in intensity and we had broken the back bone of the sudden influx of casualties, as many nurses as possible were sent on leave. This time we were not recalled. Although spared from long hours we were not spared from the bombings made over London.

After a couple of day's rest, I went to Broadcasting House as promised. Blithly alighting from the train at Oxford Circus, I walked confidently straight into Broadcasting House, showed my pass, and as I was half way through the inner gates, simultaneously, a camera flashed, and the heavy hand of a policeman grabbed my shoulder.

"Where do you think you're going?" he admonished.

"I had intended visiting my old colleagues in the news room, until you stopped me. What have I done wrong?" I enquired.

To my bewilderment he answered "Nothing."

"Well why can't I go in?" I enquired again.

"You can go in little lady, when King Haakon has left" he said with a smile.

Feeling like a naughty child I waited with the policeman, until this exceptionally tall, regal gentleman had left the building. During my two months at Broadcasting House while awaiting my call up, I also saw Queen Whilhemena. One could only admire the Royalty, who spared themselves nothing in an effort to keep in constant touch with their own people. Often ignoring a heavy bombing raid to broadcast at regular intervals across the English Channel.

My leave went all too quickly, but it was interesting to return to Haslar. Reporting for duty on a Sunday morning, one patient in a wheel chair wanted to go to church. Getting permission from Sister to take him, I wheeled him along the corridors to the lovely little chapel. On arrival we found it already packed with patients, but we were within earshot, and I knew that he had derived a lot of joy from being able to go.

Within a few days fourteen of us were notified that we were on draft to the Royal Naval Hospital Woolton. I felt rather sad to leave Haslar, as the hole in the fence had been very handy, and I had learned that if you wanted to go to a dance, it was exciting to go to bed, fully dressed, and to slip out after lights out, and trust to luck that you didn't get caught sneaking in. If Madam ever knew of our pranks I do not know, but when she saw us off on draft, I could only feel admiration for her too, and the many other titled Ladies who had given up an entirely different way of life to put wholeheartedly their time into a war-time occupation. Some of whom became just V.A.D.s like us all, and performed the same duties, and worked the same hours, literally becoming one of us, their true identity often unknown.

Travelling all day from Portsmouth in as miserable a wet, cold, and foggy day as it possibly could be, we did little else but read and talk casually to one another. Only one of my companions had I seen at Haslar.

Pouring rain and fog and a naval van greeted us at 8 p.m. on Liverpool Station. Together with our baggage, we organised ourselves in the back of the van. After being driven around for about half an hour, we landed up in a cemetry. Bit early I thought, as the driver admitted he had lost the way. Starting all over again we eventually arrived at our new hospital.

WOOLTON

Alighting from the back of the van the large grey silhouette, we could only just distinguish in the merest suggestion of grey light, that seemed to filter through from nowhere, and gave the impression of a huge monastery.

As the door opened our new Matron welcomed us. With only the aid of her torch, we all groped along a dark, long stony corridor to the mess room, where a hot cup of tea, and fish cakes were awaiting us.

So far there were only a couple of Sisters and a few other nurses and as yet no patients.

This huge building set in magnificent grounds had been previously used as an aged people's home. It was very badly in need of a good scrubbing out, and to our dismay, all windows had been covered with black paint instead of proper black out curtains. Being the first few nurses drafted to Woolton, we had to set to work with the Sisters and prepare the whole place to receive patients.

After a very long tiring journey, and supper over, this bedtime story didn't deter a really good night's sleep. For weeks

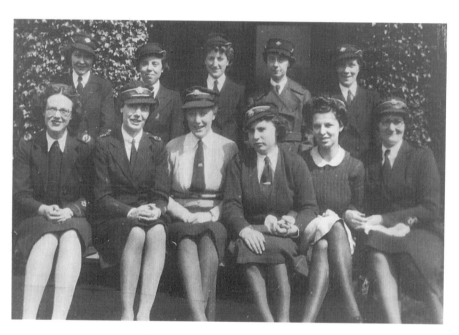

A group of the first V.A.Ds to arrive at Woolton.

with ladders, buckets, scrubbing brushes and plenty of elbow grease, we scrubbed, scoured, scraped and scratched until our very homely little hospital began to shine. Gradually streak by streak made with our razor blades, the sun filtered through the queer patterns we made on the windows, until they shone with a final polish. The morgue was renovated and transformed into our lovely little sitting room.

The building was laid out like an enormous E. One end, which was three storied was transformed into wards M1, 2 and 3. The other end became wards F1, which was the offender's ward, F2 was the wren's ward and F3 was to become the V.A.D.s quarters. The mess which was used by both nurses and patients, centred the lay-out beneath our rec-room. Only white screens petitioned our mess tables from the patients. Opposite the mess hall were the kitchens.

Small wards for officers ran along the corridors from the mess hall towards the men's wards. M1, was made up of three very large rooms and catered for medical cases. M2 was also made up of three very large rooms and was surgical. M3, only had two large rooms, one for gastric patients and the other for T.B. The wren's ward cared for all disabilities as did F1. Matron's office and the dispensary were placed along the corridor between the mess hall and the wren's ward. The operating theatre situated next to our sitting room, was half way down towards M2.

The whole atmosphere gave one a feeling of belonging to an oversized family in an oversized home, rather than a hospital. The thrill and enthusiasm of taking part in cleaning and turning an old place into a spotlessly clean one, and to see it taking shape was more like preparing a home for ourselves. Before we had finished, our first patients began to arrive, and so a couple of the nurses gave up their cleaning jobs to become nurses once again.

We were very, very short of dressings and instruments, and often had to wait until the only available instruments, which were being used on another ward were finished with and sterilized, before we could do our dressings. Gradually as we were able to get more and more equipment, more and more patients arrived, until we were all absorbed into nursing duties again.

Among our first patients was one who had been blinded by bomb blast. Each day following his operation we were all waiting for the day when his bandages would be removed. With so few patients, we all took an interest in them whether we were on their ward or not. It was a very great thrill for us to know, he could distinquish light from dark, when they were first removed. Each day he progressed slowly, until his sight was fully restored.

My first duty was on M1, now almost filled with patients, one of whom had been under observation and was to be transferred to the main hospital at Seaforth for a major operation. We were only an annexe of Seaforth, and all major cases were not held by us, although many operations were performed in our own theatre. "If you wouldn't mind, would you repair my pyjamas before I leave" he asked me as his others had not returned from the laundary. Granting his request and after returning them to him he handed me a letter before going on to Seaforth. Simply and sincerely thanking me in writing, he added a p.s. don't forget to say a little prayer for me. This took me by surprise. Such a simple job, such a simple request, I hoped his operation was a success as I never heard of him again.

News came through that my mother had been very ill. How I wished I could see her for just a short while. Two years had passed since I had seen any of them, and although I had completely resigned myself to waiting a good deal longer yet, the urge to go home was sapping my enthusiasm of resignation. My father was still trying to arrange somehow to get me home, and in the event of his being able to do so, I requested permission for my release. To my surprise it was granted, and it was now up to me to do all I could to find some way of speeding up my return home. I had exhausted all avenues I could think of and waited for hope in an unknown direction as yet.

Work in the hospital soon began to speed up, and more and more nurses and Sisters began to arrive to swell our ranks. Joy was one of them, and we were to become firm friends and share many escapades. We were fortunate in having our day and night duties to coincide with each other, and the same off duty times. I somehow feel there was great consideration there on someone's part. Day duty, night duty and mess duties alternated month by month. It wasn't long before I was on F2. A hop, skip and thud from F3 and you were on duty. For some unknown reason one of my wren patients seemed to develop a form of hero worship for me, and followed me from bed to bed whenever the opportunity presented itself. Each time I went off duty, she made me promise to see her as soon as I came on duty again. She was also very persistent that I should visit her home and meet her mother and father when she went on sick leave. Realizing somewhat sadly that she was very lonely, I promised her I would as soon as I had a free weekend, as she lived reasonably handy to Liverpool.

The promised weekend duly arrived and off I went, but was very saddened to see the humble, cramped semi-slum flat, she and her family lived in. How I wished I could take her home with me, and put her on a horse's back and let her ride free, happily surrounded by sheep that were being mustered for sheering, with their incessant plaintive bleating, only being broken by the occasional bark of an efficient sheep dog. Or to

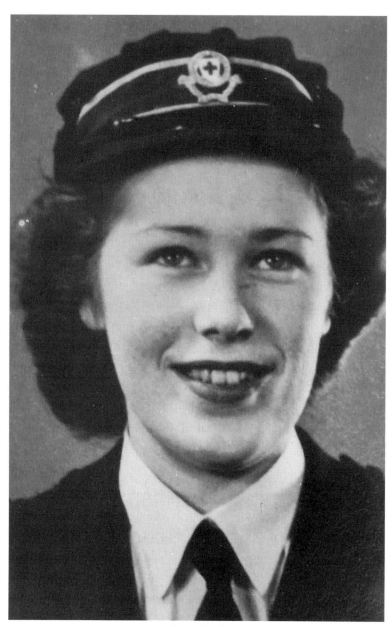

Lovely Joy

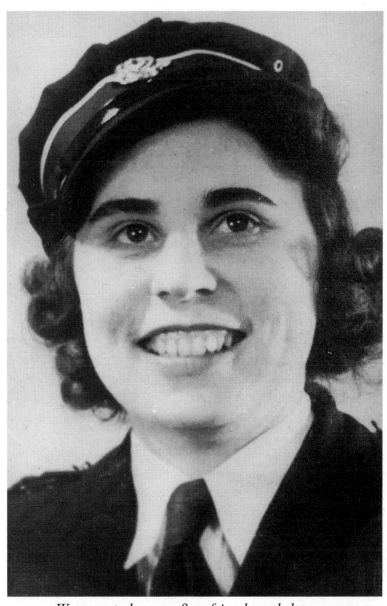

We were to become firm friends and share many escapades.

watch a busy farmer herding in his cows for milking and listen to the throbbing of the milking machines as he approached the milking sheds, and yes even to hear an irate farmer displaying his versatility of cow-shed language, on his over anxious working dog.

I would have loved to have given her a big push, and then followed her into the rolling surf of one of our many many beaches, and let her be carefree and race up and down sand dunes, or absorb the magificent enchanting serene beauty of our acres and acres of native virgin bush. To motor through Waipoua forest, and gaze up to the sky at our giant kauri. To see the spectacular rata proudly exhibiting its brilliant red flowers as it entwined itself around anything in its path. The majestic rimu, or our exotic pohutukawa, known as New Zealand's Christmas tree, that lines miles of our lovely shores bursting into a vivid splash of scarlet every Christmas, or just the smell of our homely pine, whose cones make superb firing. If in luck to hear the tranquil silvery note of our bell bird, or to watch our friendly and loveable fan-tail flitting in amongst the rich gold of the kowhai.

To fill her heart with delight, I would have loved to have taken her to a Maori concert, to see the smooth natural flowing rhythm of a poi dance and to hear the fascinating soft swishing tempo of the piupiu while the dancers are in motion. The amazing skilful handling of a long poi. The spirited, rousing, stirring haka, echoed by an infectious chorus of Maori entertainers. To meet our Maori people, whose very depth of sincerity, simplicity and natural respect for others, whose high intelligence gives our country its tradionally amazing culture. Their very disposition would cheer anyone's heart.

But these things she would never experience, and no doubt would live out her life, in her seemingly cramped way, right there in St. Helens. "Mum, dad, this is Kiwi," suddenly brought me back to earth. Having made it my business, to live and work and associate with as much of England's various classes of people during my stay there, I felt very much at home. Accepting and appreciating their very kind hospitality, I promised to return one day.

Before leaving I was given a gift of a pair of solid glass swans, blown especially for me, by her father who was a glass blower. This made me feel very humble, as I felt I had only extended friendship to a rather lonely wren, and treasure those swans still.

Back on duty on Monday morning I found we had a new nurse, who reminded me of a very beautiful flower. She was obviously well bred and well educated, and quite unaccustomed to the many chores we now took in our stride. Leaving her to watch the milk, and cook an egg for a gastric patient I continued on with one of the million other jobs that had to be done. Popping in to see how she was getting on, I overheard her politely asking Sister how you knew when the egg was cooked.

"Prick it with a fork," Sister smiled.

"Sister!" I chuckled as I walked in and we all burst into contagious and uncontrolled laughter. We really did have an inexperienced nurse with us, but she took it all in good fun, and accepted every heart-breaking and less glamourous task in her own happy refined style adding to the cheerful co-operative atmosphere that was our good fortune to enjoy.

"Nurse would you check the d.c.l." Sister asked. I discovered with shock that our d.c.l. (dangerous case list) had done irreparable damage by a self-induced abortion, causing herself much suffering and almost her life. Never having come in contact with such sordid degradation before, it grieved me very deeply that anyone could so abuse a God given privelege. Each day her young naval husband was able to visit her, and they seemed devoted to one another. As the days went by, and

41

she came off the d.c.l. and her temperature began to drop, I asked her whatever made her do it. "Oh nurse, we love each other and don't want any children," she proudly explained. Dumbfounded I could not understand why a young married woman could do such a thing, but under stress of circumstances one could perhaps understand a young single girl fearing untimely and vicious critisism from those who should at least help her over her own mental suffering and consider the unborn child. Back in the cabin I thought of Norma who had recently married and had realized she was expecting before her Army husband had been posted overseas. She was a very broken-hearted patient who had lost her infant. Neither of them knowing when her husband would return, but hoping together it would be their turn next time. Norma's sincerity impressed me and I heard from her often after her discharge.

I was not sorry when off duty time came that day, and slowly mounted the stairs to our quarters. As I went into our over crowded room, taking my cap off as I did so, I wondered what had happened to Sylvia as she walked around the dorm, with a hot water bottle sitting on her head. Obviously thinking I thought she was nuts, "I've washed my hair and I'm trying to get it dry for the dance tonight" she smiled.

"Oh yes I'm going, I'd forgotten," I remembered verbally. By the time I had polished all my buttons and insignias on my out door uniform, and we had had competitions in seeing who could make what we called the smartest fowls' bottoms which we had nick-named our caps, and we were ready to go early in the evening, the day's tragedy had passed from my mind. With gay abandon a crowd of us went together laughing and chatting as we walked to accept the invitation that had been extended to us.

"Are you the N.F.S.?" we were asked by the guards on the gate as we approached.

"No, the B.R.C.S.!" unexpectedly came from me, surprising me with a wit I didn't know I had. Laughingly he opened the gate for us, and we soon found ourselves in a small very smokey room, and offered a welcoming drink as a prelude to joining the already crowded floor.

As I had no taste for drink the insistence to continue drinking became rather boring. Finally giving up in favour of dancing my airman partner compromised by remarking, "You have such lovely eyes. They have that beautiful far away look."

Not being accustomed to his obviously artificial flattery I felt my cheeks flush and chuckingly replied, "Yes I know, thirteen thousand miles away!" This brought no relief.

"Are they all as beautiful as you in New Zealand?" he tried again. This was the end.

"No" I replied. "Much better!" and dodged away as soon as opportunity presented itself. Joining in with the other dancers, to the tunes of *'Don't Sit Under the Apple Tree,'* and *'Doing the Lambeth Walk'* and many others, the evening passed all too quickly.

Walking home, Joy and I planned how we would get in unseen as it was well past midnight. Deciding to cut around the side of the hospital hoping the side door on the corridor by the kitchens was unlocked, we stumbled and groped in the darkness through the trees that flanked our hospital, giggling helplessly each time we slipped on the moss covered stones, for fear of being heard if we laughed outright. Halfway round I slipped and cut my leg. Eventually arriving and finding the side door unlocked, we slipped in, and the dim light in the corridor, enabled us to see the blood dripping from my leg. There was just too much not to report. Joy stayed with me as we silently tip-toed to the receiving office, hoping the S.B.A. on duty was sporting. To our horror the Senior Medical Officer was in the cabin. Caught wasn't the word, and we knew it was no good trying to get out of it. As he dressed the rather deep cut he questioned us on how it happened. Still in happy mood I told him. "Why didn't you come in the main door?" he questioned. Sheepishly looking at Joy I told him, we didn't want to get caught coming in so late. Quietly smiling to himself, "Well don't cut your leg the next time, will you?" With a sigh of relief Joy and I crept up happily to our quarters, with thumping hearts each time we heard footsteps, in case we were caught in the corridors.

Having morning tea the next day sitting on the couch in our sitting-room, I was suddenly overcome with an overtaking feeling of utter exhaustion and nausea. Fortunately I was able to control it's determined insistence, until the next batch of nurses appeared for morning-tea. Miserably requesting a hasty bowl, it arrived in just the nick of time. "You'll have to report to sick-bay," I was advised. "She's right, it'll soon pass," but it was no good, as I felt so much on fire, and a very sharp pain in my side took command of the whole situation. Capitulating under my protests, it was very peaceful to be resting in the ward I was on duty on half an hour before. As soon as the doctor had left, I learned that I had a grumbling appendix.

"Blow that for a joke," I remarked. "It's not grumbling it's doing a haka!" brought an amused smile from Sister as she left me to my thoughts. Reflecting on minus one appendix, liquid diet and being just a lady I caught up on some of the sleep I had so happily missed the night before.

Next morning I felt a real fake, as my temperature had dropped and the pain had gone. I was discharged when the doctor had been. Simply slipping upstairs to put on my indoor uniform, I descended the stairs again. Sister had sent me on escort duty, as there had been an accident and the V.A.D. (Voluntary Aid Detachment) had fainted after all the experience we had had, surely it must be some accident. As the ambulance sped along in the grey miserable mist rain with a skilful driver, miraculously negotiating the sharp turns and slippery roads, I was jolted from side to side, while I went over in my head; first arrest any haemorrhage, treat for shock, and above all don't faint yourself. Boosting my confidence with my self-administered good advice, we rolled into an effortless stop. Stepping out into a cold unpleasant drizzle, I crossed the street and knocked on a cafe door, and was politely shown into a cosy, compact, well lit back room. It was simply but pleasantly furnished, with a large dining table, four chairs, and a couch alongside a warm inviting fire.

Leaning with her elbows on the table, was an elderly pleasant woman gently talking to a V.A.D. driver, whose forehead was cupped in one hand, as she sipped a cup of tea with the other. "Where is the patient? I enquired

"There," smiled our hostess.

"But I thought there had been an accident?" I enquired again.

"Yes, the ambulance skidded and hit a lamp post and the V.A.D. driver fainted, so I brought her in here, gave her a warm drink, and rang the hospital to let someone know." Wryly smiling at my easy let out of an anticipated busy morning's work, I accepted with gratitude a very welcome cup of tea, as I knew I had dipped out on one by this time, and then left with our patient who had almost recovered from her shock.

Settling in the back of the ambulance our patient who was usually a very bright and sparkling personality, very demurely apologized for having caused such a stir. "I only wish all accidents were as pleasant as this" I answered her knowing how embarrassed she must have felt, as we returned to the hospital at a much easier speed.

The doctor we had with us, who had travelled with the driver considerately invited us into the ward-room for a drink as it was so cold and miserable outside. Amidst congenial chaffing while sipping a glass of very beautiful wine, we were soon all sparkling again. As my patient returned to her quarters for a rest, I returned to my ward wishing all emergencies could end so happily.

Typically calmly Sister asked what I had done with the patient. Smiling I whispered, "Smell my breath."

With dancing eyes and bewilderment she remarked "What have you been up to, I wish I had gone!"

Escort duties seemed always to come in runs. Afternoon tea brought my off duty time. While I was at tea, one of my Wren patients who had been wheeled in a wheel chair by another patient to afternoon tea, offered me some home made shortbread, which had been sent to her by her mother in Scotland. It was an unexpected joy to me. A few minutes later, she called me again in a very feeble voice and was almost in a state of collapse. She wanted only me to take her back to the ward. I had to wheel her very slowly as the movement made her feel very ill. Back on the ward two of us very gently put her into bed. "Stay with me Kiwi," was all she could say. I stayed till she settled, although I was officially off duty an hour previously. I waited till she felt she would be alright as she was vomiting continously.

When a lull came I asked her if I could go and promised to be with her as soon as I came on duty next morning. "I'll be alright now," she very feebly answered. I did not like to leave her as I felt so uneasy about her.

Before I reached the top of the stairs to our quarters, I heard Sister say, "Send Nurse Plane." Somehow I knew I would not see her again.

As I heard someone mounting the stairs calling me, fear gripped me, and I slipped into the night nurse's quarters, continuing to give them the slip until they returned to the ward. From the small window in the toilet about half an hour later, I saw the ambulance drive away. As it drove off, I turned only half conscious of my surroundings, and for some unknown reason despondently dressed to go ashore. As I passed the Wren's ward on my way out, one of my colleagues, astonished to see me, exclaimed "We've been looking all over for you to escort a patient to the morgue." A cold shudder went through me as I knew who it was without asking.

It was a great relief to be off duty. Joy and I went to the quiet club in Liverpool to relax to some of the very wide range of recordings, that were at anyone's disposal. It was a quiet club, consisting of reading and writing rooms, and small sound proof music rooms. Wanting to cheer myself up, I selected *'Espana.'* After it had repeated itself several times Joy became impatient and threatened to lift the needle if it repeated itself again. It did, so she carried out her threat and replaced my record with *'Madam Butterfly.'*

Half way through her recording I returned her impatience with mine, and laughingly we decided to go to a favourite haunt of ours. Walking to Sissons for an excellent bun and cup of tea, we were accompanied by a recording of Vera Lynn singing *'Concerto for Two'* through loud speakers over the streets.

At a bit of a loss to know what to do we went to see *"For Whom the Bell Tolls"* and finished off by going to Penny Lane Canteen. Finding a couple of empty chairs, we were puzzled when Joy was offered two match sticks. The wise cracking that persisted with our ignorance, was soon drowned out by some unaccomplished serviceman thumping out *'Roll out the Barrel'* on an old cigarette stained piano, which was almost passed retuning. God bless the unpolished pianist who braved the chidings and noisy raggings everytime he hit a wrong note, but gave us many a very happy evening. It was always fun to try to pick from the many accents, which part of the country they had come from, and just as much fun to be wrong every time. The Irish accent fascinated me, and so did the Scotch, because mostly I couldn't understand it at all.

Returning on duty next morning, one of my patients wanted to go to church. Being Sunday morning we only had a skeleton staff. This could have been difficult but it did not deter Sister Marsden whose placid but happy nature always had a solution. She never ever became ruffled and suggested I take her. She would have been on her own, but her nurses and patients always came first. During her training days she had performed a tracheotomy with a pen knife on a small child in an ambulance on her way to a hospital, and thus saved his life. When we were ready to leave I asked my patient which church she wanted to go to. We had quite a long walk, and I had to stay with her all the time as she could not be left on her own. On our return she gave me a clipping she had found in a magazine, and it was so full of sincerity, that like my swans I treasure it too.

That afternoon was so cold and wet, that to remain in the hospital did not appeal when I came off duty. Instead I went to the Liverpool Philharmonic Hall, to see and hear Doctor Malcolm Sargeant conducting the Liverpool Philharmonic Orchestra. Before each orchestral piece was played, he explained its story, which made the whole afternoon most interesting and worthwhile. Every Sunday afternoon these lovely concerts were held. In uniform it only cost us 6d. to sit behind the orchestra. The first time I went I was nearly deafened by the huge drum in front of me. I soon got wise to this and found that it paid to be late, so that all those seats would be filled, and still get in at 6d. and sit in the front row of the hall itself.

Soon my month on F 2 came to a close and I found myself back on M 1 Just as I was about to descend the stairs, Betty hailed me from the stairs on her way up to M 3 "Hey Kiwi what's a goose neck?" This question brought hilarious laughter from the M 2 patients.

"I've never heard of it!" I called back and carried on to M 1 When we did find out, we hoped we would not get on to M 2 for some time.

M 1 had changed greatly since I was last on duty there. One of the three wards was full of V.D. patients. Not the most pleasant type of patient to nurse, but nevertheless they required nursing, and who are we to judge the misdemeanours of others. On the whole they were no different from any other patient, but one always had an instinctive reserve in the form of conversation with them. Very few were proud of their misfortunes but one young lad in his early twenties openly bragged of his sordid associations in brothels around the world, mocking at those who were too proud to be natural according to his way of life. Suffering greatly for his ignorance, he was waiting for the day when he would be discharged for the third time, to be able to enjoy life again. It wasn't very pleasant working in that atmosphere, but one had to accept it as, 'it takes all sorts to make a world'. Perhaps he needed mental care rather than medical.

Across the small hall that separated the wards, was a rather quiet, decent type of lad, who had jaundice from the treatment for V.D.

One afternoon while giving him his medicine, "You don't like me Kiwi" he very quietly ventured. Sensing he was rather broken over something, I quietly told him, as far as I knew there was only one way to contract the disease but there were exceptions. With tears not far away, he told me he had got it from his wife who had been entertaining a wide variety of companions while he had been away at sea for many months.

Frozen with horror, at first I could not believe any woman could indulge in such disloyal practices while her husband was overseas. As time went on I heard of so many who had lived up to the reputation of a certain type of sailor with a wife in every port.

On fine days, as we were on ground level two nurses had to lift strict bed patients on to the lawn, beds and all, as we had no men to help us. The war was gaining in intensity, and for half an hour a week all patients and staff had to wear gas masks. This was no joke and extremely uncomfortable. One morning while working in our gas masks I was fortunate in seeing the arms of a heart case drop by his sides. Unhesitantly I slipped his gas mask off and raised his shoulders on to his pillows, but as I felt for his pulse, he gripped my hand without even opening his eyes or making any other movement. I just remained there, greatly relieved his heart was still beating. After some time he slowly opened his eyes, as he turned his head in my direction, "God bless you Kiwi, you saved my life," he very slowly voiced. "One day when I'm well I'm going to visit your lovely country again and walk you through Lyttleton Tunnel," he smiled to me. "Two of us did it many years ago, we went in white one end, and came out pitch black the other!" he told me. Almost speechless from relief to see him able to tease again, I told him I did not feel I had done that at all, as any other nurse would have done the same. I continued to talk of how one day I would get home again and hoped he would visit me if he ever got there too.

As I was leaving his bedside, the patient next to him asked me to post a letter for him. Having sealed it, he crossed the bottom of the flap, putting an initial in three of the spaces. As he handed it to me he said, "There used to be four of us, but my young daughter of four was killed in a raid." The horrors of war were really spreading its sadistical tentacles.

Time seemed to slip by very quickly on that ward, with a large number of patients coming and going. Most of our patients had been replaced by a very happy crowd, whose wit cheered the whole atmosphere. On my last afternoon before my stand-off, prior to going on night duty, I was called by a

50

patient into the sluice-room. Unsuspecting I went to see what was wanted. Very politely three of them faced me and explained I could not go on nights without learning how to give a blanket-bath properly. Dumped clothes and all into the bath, I received a detailed lecture and demonstration with the aid of sand soap and a scrubbing brush. All my protests were ignored by extra scrubs. With a limp dripping cap and the back of my uniform soaked, it was not easy to slip up the stairs, pass M 2, along the full length of all the corridors, pass F 2, as well as all the day staff till I reached the safety of our quarters to change my uniform. Not to mention jolly sore arms and legs.

Late that afternoon when Joy came off duty we went for a stroll. Woolton canteen was very restful after a tiring day's work. There was usually someone playing table tennis, and the few that went there found relaxation over a cup of tea. One evening as Joy and I sauntered in, more asleep than awake, we were enchanted by the strains of very beautiful music coming from the canteen. As we entered we found an airman lost in his piano playing. When he stopped the canteen seemed dead. Neither Joy nor I had the courage to ask him to carry on. As he remained seated at the piano, the urge was too great, so I went over to request *'Ave Maria'*. He turned, and once again beauty filled the canteen. "Any other tune you would like?" he asked. Opportunities like this were too good to miss, so I requested *'The Rustle of Spring'*.

This type of piano playing was very rare, and I just couldn't help remarking "You play well enough for a gifted pianist."

"I have my cap and gown in music, but only play for pleasure," he returned, and then joined us in a cup of tea. We went again to enjoy the unselfish talent of this airman, but learned to our very great disppointment that he had been posted.

51

CHRISTMAS AND NEW HOPE

Christmas was fast approaching. There is something extra beautiful about Christmas in England. It not only has an air of festivity and gaity, but also a deep reverence enhanced by the ringing of church bells and carols from carillons. The hoped for pure white carpet of freshly fallen snow creates a feeling of purity, and one could almost feel, they too were reborn each Christmas, and all thoughts seemed to be mutual, with a good will towards all with whom one associated.

The beautiful services and joyous celebrations annually marking the birth of our Saviour, must each year renew friendships and bring together many who otherwise may be forgotten. This first Christmas at Woolton was to become a very memorable one for me.

Toni, who was a member of the St. John ambulance, did much to capture the solemnity and beauty of this happy season. She had a set of beautifully toned hand bells, and arranged for five of us to get together to learn to play some of the loveliest carols. The music was written in numbers on the music sheet: every moment we could get together we practiced till we were able to handle the bells properly.

On Christmas Eve, with freshly starched caps and fresh crisp white aprons, we wore our capes inside out, so that the inner red lining was outside. With dimmed lights in all wards and along the corridors, we played continously as we went from ward to ward and slowly along the corridors.

'Silent Night', loved the world over, played with feeling on Toni's bells, must have touched the hearts of all who heard them, and brought that inner feeling of peace and hope, for a short time, to forget the harsh realities and sufferings of war.

Christmas time was not holiday time during the war and I soon found myself on night's on M1. I only hoped the patients that were so full of pranks were not still on the ward. The report book showed one patient had to be watched, as he had had a blood transfusion for anaemia. All was peace and quiet, with one patient complaining with mirth, that they gave the cow too much water to drink. The senior nurse he told me was so efficient she wandered around like Nelson.

With the last light switched off and the after-thought wise-cracking had faded into the dark and stillness of night, I was attracted by an unusual strange sound coming from the sluice-room. Puzzled, I went to investigate. To my amusement and delight, I found the bottom of the bath filled with about two dozen frogs with sufficient water to keep them happy. I spent some time lining them up and seeing which one could win a race to the other end of the bath. Quietly enjoying myself, but as they persisted in jumping their own ways and not observing any rules of the game I left them to it. Passing through the bathroom and sluice-room, I was confronted with almost every patient peeping around the door. "What on earth......" I faultered.

"We've been waiting for you to scream, Nurse!" they announced together.

"Too bad!" I returned. "Frogs fascinate me and they'll make great playmates when I am stuck for something to do in the middle of the night. They are supposed to be the nearest creature to man. Get into bed before Sister comes," I advised them and happily continued on to the cabin to catch up on my correspondence and mending.

As I settled down, smiling to myself I became aware of a thud, and then thud again, very gently coming from nowhere. Disregarding it I began writing and again thud, thud broke the silence. Concentrating on the direction I thought it had come from, my eyes fell on an upturned bowl. Cautiously raising it, out hopped two more frogs. It's just as well I am not afraid of them placidly crossed my mind as I chased them all over the cabin until I caught them and put them back into the damp grass outside.

The following night one of the patients was very abusive. His language was uncalled for and unnecessary. Requesting him to keep it to himself as I had no desire to report him, seemed only to release a hidden aggression that was not very comfortable and caused the other patients to become disturbed. Against my will, I had to report him. He was due for discharge the following morning and had all his gear packed alongside his bed, together with his rifle. I was very uneasy about it and reported it to Sister when she came on her rounds. "Don't worry about it Nurse," was all she quite unconcernedly replied.

I had never in my life had such a solitary mental struggle to overcome the concern I felt. Never once did I dare to remove it for fear of being abused again and perhaps physically. The strain grew more and more tense as the night wore on, and every movement filled me with fear. Reading or writing became an impossibility and I longed for the dawn. As I did my rounds I was glad to leave his ward. After an endless night, the depressing dark gave way to the first light of dawn, bringing with it the gradual relief of the tension I felt. Taking round the routine temperature tray, as I passed his bed, quite cheerfully he remarked, "How do you feel this morning nurse?"

"Fine thanks but I was a bit worried about your gun."

"There was nothing to worry about it's not loaded," he casually replied.

Finishing a month of nights on M1, it was quite a break to find I was due for mess duties. After a couple of hours sleep, I dressed to go ashore. There was a concert on at the Quiet Club that I wanted to go to. Joy was on duty and usually I remained aboard when this happened, but this time I decided to go alone. The concert was well worth going to, but on coming out to my horror it was almost pitch black. Without wasting time, I went to the nearest tram stop and waited under the dimmed light of a chemist shop, which cast an eerie haze on all surroundings. Every tram except mine seemed to rumble up, stop, and rumble on again. While I was waiting there, a rather uncouth middle aged man in civvies, with a trilby pulled down well over his forehead, paced back and forth. Quite a common occurance, but each time he passed me, he came a little closer till I began to feel wary. A strange foreboding overtook me, so I boarded the next tram that rumbled up the road and changed at the next stop. Back at the hospital I related my uncanny story to Joy, and gave us both the spooks. The following morning the headlines of the newspapers carried the horrifying news, that a WAAC had been stabbed outside the chemist's shop, under the light, by an unknown man in a trilby hat. I shuddered, had my ever faithful guardian angel warned me of this impending danger. Never again would I go out alone.

A message had been left at the hospital, that a New Zealander had called while I was out and left a phone number for me to ring. This really was intriguing, and I wasted no time to solve the mystery. On my next afternoon off I met him in Liverpool and he took me to the Empire Rendezvous. There were many New Zealanders there. The presence of Kiwis touched off a great patriotic pride I never knew I had. I had never known a greater joy than that afternoon just simply talking to many who had so recently been in New Zealand. "You must see Bill, he'll get you home," they cheerfully encouraged. "If he doesn't we will!" gave me a great lift and at least some hope and more avenues to try. News had come through that my mother had been in hospital; how I wished I had some way I could see her for just a short while. Once again I wrote to Red Cross headquarters but could only draw a blank. So I discussed it with our matron and senior medical officer and they offered to do all they could to help me.

Mess duties was always a very cheerful break, as one was spared the saddening contact of treating severe wounds inflicted in combat. The recovering patients morale commanded great admiration.

One patient was nicknamed Nelson, as he had lost an eye and an arm. He was so full of fun and energy that he had been threatened that if he broke his fifth eye replacement, he would not get anymore. Every afternoon sharp on 3pm, Jock came down to the mess room on his artificial leg. "Hello Kiwi what's the time?" he asked in his broad Scotch accent every time.

One afternoon I beat him to it "Have you come to see me again Jock?" I called out as I heard him coming.

"Oh no Kiwi, just to see the time," he answered back.

"Am I allowed to ask what you did with your other leg?" I asked him.

"I left it under a train," he took me by surprise. "I can't blame the war for that," he explained. "I came right through Dunkirk without a scratch and when we got back, all of us who were sent home on leave, celebrated on the train to

Scotland and I got so drunk, I walked off the train, and my leg went under the wheel and I don't know where it is now." Quite unconcerned and happy he returned to his ward.

While the patients drifted in one lunch time, one with a particularly good physique casually withdrew a chair and placed it alongside one of the long mess tables. Thoughtfully placing his two hands on the chair back, he slowly raised his entire body off the floor until it was in a horizontal position, and then carried on to a vertical position. Giving a quick flip, he released the chair and landed upright on his feet.

Going off duty to change and go ashore, I walked into great hilarity. There had been a notice on the board, 'Would Venus please refrain from parading in front of the V.A.D.s windows.' We had become accustomed to the only two V.A.D.s I ever came across who had lost their self-respect somewhere in their upbringing, but with the patients on the M wards complaining as our quarters were directly opposite, it ceased.

Arriving at the Empire Rendezvous, it was very amazing to be asked if I wanted to buy an overcoat by some Kiwis. "Blue's run out of beer money and wants to sell his clothes to get some more!" Only laughter answered that one. Collecting a plate of sausages and mash, and trying to do justice to it, I was whisked away to meet Bill. There, surrounded by jovial Kiwis, in his well known thick horn rimmed glasses, was our own beloved Bill Jordan, New Zealand's High Commissioner in London.

"Look Bill we found a lost Kiwi that wants to get home," was my introduction.

Sitting me on his knee like a small child, he asked for my story. After relating it, like the grand person he was, "I'll be your father while you're in England, you must come and visit my wife whenever you come to London. Write to me at my office and I'll do my best for you, but I can't make any promises," he told me. Filled with greater hope I returned to the hospital.

There was a concert on in the rec-room put on by the staff. Their skit of an operation being performed behind a sheet so that we could only see their shadows, kept the hall full of laughter. Plaster cast legs and arms being sawn off and thrown aside, a huge hammer to quieten the patient while they removed yards and yards of sausages for his appendix, kept everyone laughing.

That weekend Joy and I had sleeping out passes. On the invitation from her father, he drove us to their home. Because I had never been through it, he took us through the world famous Mersey Tunnel on our way to Anglesey in North Wales. Stopping half way to their home, he took us to a hotel for dinner, where the atmosphere was so peaceful and quiet after the communal way of life we had become accustomed to. At Joy's home, it was almost a dream to sit and chat quietly in a cosy sitting room with the luxury of a fire. The following morning Joy took me for a walk around a beautiful little Welsh village, stopping and talking to all she knew. Their soft Welsh voices and language added to the beauty of that lovely village, still with some of its quaint little houses. What a very beautiful place Anglesey was, and what a lovely rest we had. Her parents were so kind to me that I was sorry when the weekend was over.

Reluctantly returning to the hospital, I wrote to Mr. Jordan, keeping my fingers crossed.

For a change Joy and I decided to go to a dance at the Anzac Club, which was opposite the Empire Redezvous. Going up in the lift and booking in our coats at the cloak room, we ventured into the dance hall. Before we had time to look around, we were swept on to the floor by two Chinese men. As they danced they carried on a conversation in Malay. When the music stopped I simply said "tidak" which meant no in Malay. They both stared at one another as though stupified.

"You speak Malay?" one enquiringly faltered.

"Yes," I replied confidently.

"You know what we talk about?"

"Every word," I answered, which was an exaggeration, but I had remembered sufficient to pick up the undesirable intentions they had in mind.

"You speak Chinese too?" he questioned.

"No," I answered.

"You come to my flat I teach you," he slyly smiled.

"No thanks," I told him and as soon as we were out of ear shot, Joy and I slipped out unseen. As soon as the coast was clear, we collected our coats and went quickly into the open lift, breathing a sigh of relief as the gates closed and we descended below. Alighting from the lift we were startled to find the two Chinese waiting for us on the ground floor. How they knew we were leaving I do not know.

"I walk you home," they adamantly insisted. We were trapped and we knew it. I do not remember how we gave them the slip, but by changing trams frequently and almost running out of money we eventually arrived back at the hospital alone and never went there again.

I was due for leave and went to stay with a friend in Ilford. I hadn't seen her and her small daughter Valerie for quite some time. When I arrived, her place was locked and they were asleep. No calling or knocking stirred her. It was too cold to sleep on her doorstep till morning, so found her rubbish tin and climbed in through the open skylight in the bathroom. I searched round, made a hot drink and used all the coats I could find, and curled up on her couch to fall into a deep sleep. Next morning Jo was very alarmed to find me sound asleep. Worried as to how I got in, she was pleased to learn of the only available entrance in, that from then on she locked it. It was wonderful to hear all her news and that her husband who was away overseas in the Eighth Army was coming through his cruel combats still in one piece. He had never seen his daughter.

I learned the raids over London had intensified, and the night I had arrived was the first they'd had any respite. Exhausted by the continual bombings was why Jo had slept so soundly. Home cooked meals and no routine made my stay most enjoyable.

After a couple of days relaxation, I went to New Zealand House in London to persue my desire to get home. Mr. Jordon was still away visiting New Zealanders wherever they were, but I was invited to take part in a broadcast home the following day. This was a great thrill to look forward to. Back at Jo's we discussed what I would say in the few minutes each New Zealander had to send a message home.

That night all hell was let loose. Being a V.A.D. I had to notify the Police where I was staying in case I was needed. Bombs crashed down all round us. The whole earth seemed to vibrate under the cruel explosions. Monstrous fires encircled us. Angry, vicious and terrorising. Jo's next door neighbour became hysterical and all her children screamed and cried in terror. They were very difficult to get into the maximum safety of the Morrison shelter. Fortunately Valerie had been put to bed in the shelter and slept peacefully through it all. Sleep was an utter impossibility for Jo and me. We alternated drinking tea and coffee, as every minute I was expecting to have to go on duty. To venture into the open was sheer madness even with a tin-hat on as flak was hitting the road and pavements ceaselessly. The dog-fights overhead were continuous with occasional planes dropping from the skies in flames. The ack-ack guns with their heroic crews, often young women, kept up continual fire. I gazed up at this fearful sight.

"Oh God please don't let these maniacs drop any bombs, or allow any blazing planes drop on us, to maim us, or destroy us. I need my arms and my legs to carry on the work I had grown to enjoy so much, and our hospital are so full already, and every nurse is needed." Prayer was the only real comfort we had.

When dawn broke the upheaval of the night quietened. Feeling completely exhausted I made my way to London, passing great destruction, and many fires still burning. The smell of burning human flesh was sickening, as ambulance men still worked feverishly to rescue as many casualties as they could, and removing those that had been killed. Parentless children were filthy with grime from the fires, and wandered homeless, weeping and bewildered from one demolished house to another. Screaming every now and then as they trod on a piece of smoldering wood, or hot rubble or flak.

Nauseated I finally arrived at the New Zealand club, just in time to join the rest of the party to go on to 200, Oxford St. and be met by Miss Noni Wright. An Aucklander herself, she arranged the sessions "Anzac's Calling Home". As each of us made our broadcast, we were photographed at the mike. When all messages had been recorded, we were invited to morning tea. It was rather like, being on my own home ground once again, but in a different section. We were advised that we could hear our own broadcasts being sent overseas in about a fortnight's time. This too was exciting to look forward to.

Soon my leave was over and I hated leaving Jo's. Before returning to Liverpool I called in to see another friend whose husband was a paratrooper, and had just been posted overseas. He was singing out of tune to his small daughter seated on his knee, *"You are my sunshine"*, as though expressing in his own way what he was going away to fight for. Within a fortnight he had been killed.

61

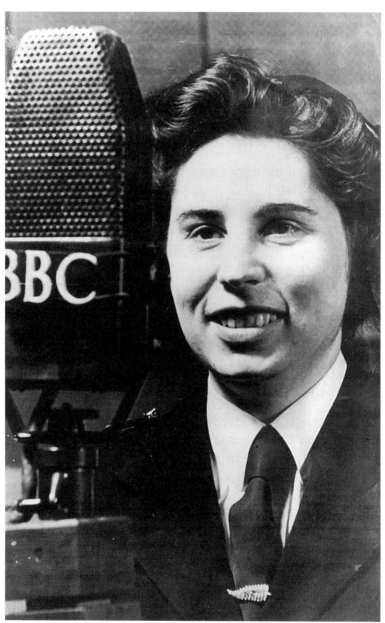

Taking part in 'Anzacs Calling Home', 1943

Returning to Woolton there was a letter from Mr. Jordon. Its contents explained that as shipping space was so limited, he could hold out no hope for my getting home just yet, but had made a note of my name and would notify me as soon as any became available. It seemed so useless, but at least I now had many friends from my own country, in the same boat as I which gave me great comfort. I also had a notice of when to listen to hear my own broadcast home. Talking to Joyce who spent her evenings after work, serving in the Empire Rendezvous, she invited me to go to her home to hear it. I was very grateful to her and arrived before seven in the morning. It came through very well, but I never knew before how much I sounded like an American over the air. It was lovely too, to share an English breakfast in comfort, in the calm generous air of an English family once again.

My next ward was M111 (3). There was not much to do in the way of dressings and treatments on that ward as most were gastric patients. All day and every day seemed to be taken up with running backwards and forwards, up and down the stairs collecting milk for them. One morning going on duty, one of my patients happily announced his donkey had had a baby in the night, and there in his hand he had made an almost perfect donkey from his handkerchief. It was a quiet happy ward, and sometimes it was hard to find something to do, instead of rushing round hoping you could get through your days work.

Returning from lunch one afternoon I found a message in the report-book to take all the temperatures on the T.B. ward, which was opposite and staffed by Sick Berth Attendants. The S.B.A. on duty had been called out to an emergency and would not be back in time to do them. Collecting the temp. tray, I went to take them as requested. I could not understand why all the patients had lined up in file on either side of the door, and down the centre of the ward. As soon as I stepped between them, one patient took my arm, and as they began singing the wedding march they made an archway of bed-pans. Having passed through the archway, I was led to a strict-bed patient and left alone. Puzzled by all this, the very ill patient told me he had watched me every time I passed the door, and if he got well would I marry him. I was very taken aback when he went on to say he did not think he would live long enough to marry anyone, but if he had someone to live for he might. The other patients had arranged the wedding march as they knew a nurse would be on that ward that afternoon, to try to cheer him, as he had lost all his people. Never in my life had I felt so humiliated and wished I could really do something for him. I felt I could only comfort him, by telling him that while I had my life and my health in this war, it was going into nursing and that I would visit him as often as I was allowed. Back in the cabin I looked up his bed-ticket and X-ray, and for the first time since I began nursing wanted to sit down and weep.

I couldn't stay at the hospital when I came off duty, so went alone in the evening to a dance in Woolton. Arriving at the hall I saw one of our nurses behind a table covered in beer bottles. "Oh my God she's drunk," stuck in my throat. "You haven't drunk all that have you?" I asked.

"Yes, Kiwi and I'm going to drink some more," she slurred.

"You can't, you're on duty tonight," I earnestly told her, feeling really concerned as she was a decent kid. After removing all the bottles from the table I began walking her back to the hospital. Getting her safely to her room, "For heaven's sake pull yourself together and get ready, I'll fill in till you come down, don't you dare let me down" I mildly admonished her. Like a scolded child, she began washing and changing, so I left her and filled in for her. When Sister came round and queried my being on the ward I simply told her I was standing in. As luck would have it she was satisfied.

After a while my colleague arrived on duty and burst into tears. "I'll never forget you for this Kiwi," she sobbed. "I don't know what's happened to me, I never drink, but somehow I wanted to drink and drink and get as drunk as I could." I stayed with her for a while, but was glad when I could get some rest.

It became necessary for us to have our own quarters, as we were very overcrowded in F111. With the extra nurses that had swelled our ranks, it was becoming very difficult for the night-staff to get any sleep. Joy and I had our beds so close together, that one blanket would have covered both of them. Our beds were jammed up against an unused fire-place, if we wanted to we could have pushed our heads up the chimney. Oh that loud speaker above our beds. Every night we turned it down, and every morning sharp on seven, it blared forth to stir us all. Who turned it up, we never knew. Besides working on the wards, we had to pack all our belongings, and were moved to the "Gables" in Menlove Ave. Each morning we had transport to take us to the hospital, so we couldn't be late or we would have to go by tram.

Having finished a month on M111, I was then sent to M11. I loved this ward, as it was surgical. Half way through my time on that ward, I managed to acquire a nasty cough, which worsened and began to sap all my energy. Going straight off duty and into bed, made no impression on it. With a three day stand-off coming up, I refused to give in. Jane was very insistent on reporting it as I began to feel so ill. Each morning I went on duty, I managed to get the job of sorting and counting the linen for the laundry. I folded some ready to go, and left a huge heap, that I rested on when no one was about. How I ever got away with staying on one job so long I'll never know. By the time my stand-off came, I could scarcely move, and was afraid to cough as the pain in my chest became so acute, and my head just spun behind by burning eyes. Getting straight into bed as I had planned for my stand-off, Jane, who was one of the other four girls I shared a room with, refused to give me any peace until she had taken my temp. Recording a dangerously high one she was off to report me to sick-bay. As she was walking out of the room I called after her, "If you report it Jane I'll never forgive you!" Obviously the sensible thing for her to do, but she gave in and promised to sneak my meals up to me, but if I had not improved by the Monday morning she would report it. So I settled on that. For the whole weekend Jane did as she said she would, and sometimes had to wait till 10 p.m. to get a hidden tea up to me. She was sure I had pleurisy, but by Monday morning my temperature had dropped, and although I felt weak, and almost afraid to breath, as my chest was so sore, I was very thankful to Jane and went on duty.

One of our patients was a man of sixty who had served in both World Wars, and through an accident had become partly paralysed, but was getting worse. He was affectionately known as old Pop, and was only able to make sounds instead of speaking. Suddenly vomiting violently over everything, three of the patients carried him into the bathroom to clean him up, but were unable to prevent an unpleasant trail for me to clean up. Poor old Pop was very upset about it, but the patients cheered him and told him they would help me. So with great gusto they sang *"You shouldn't have joined, you jolly well shouldn't have joined!"* Their happy chiding contributed much to the happy atmosphere of the ward, making my own task a cheery one.

Night duty on the mess was a welcome change. Instead of having frog races as in M1, we collected cockroaches and raced them instead. We had all got tired of re-heated meals, so one of the V.A.D.s who was friendly with a kitchen-staff wren, arranged with her to accidently leave a sack of potatoes out each night, so we had freshly fried chips every night for a month. Half way through one night, one of the V.A D.s with a self-satisfied smile on her face, waltzed through the mess hall as though she were nursing a baby. Proudly announcing she had a baby brought many wise-cracks from the few of us who were there. A baby in a Naval Hospital, just wasn't done. "I had a baby donkey given to me once, what did you get?" I chidingly remarked.

"A real one!" came the reply. After she had led us up the garden-path for some time, she told us who had had the baby. This surprised us all as the wren who had given birth had been on duty all that day in the kitchens!

I was delighted to find after my nights on the mess, I was to go back on to F.11 as on this ward one could be uninhibited and free to say whatever they wished. The mutual companionship that existed between us all, became more and more evident as the war turned in its entirety. There was talk of a landing in France soon, and we were all hoping for a change for the better. The ward was full and once again I landed an escort duty. The patient was Peggy, a wren mechanic, and after having completed a job, as she left the plane, the pilot revved his engine, hitting her with the propellor thus fracturing her spine. She had to be nursed face down, and taken in that position to Seaforth for an X-ray. Having got her into the ambulance, we found the cradle to support the blankets from resting on her back was too wide, so I had to support them with my arm. Slowly, with the canvas sides emblazoned with the Red Cross on either side, of our war-time ambulance, flapped in the cold wind, we began on our half-hour journey. Half-way there the ambulance stopped to refuel. As Peggy complained of being very thirsty, and we had no vessel for me to get her a drink in, I used the enamel bowl she had in case she vomited on the way. Although in pain, she thought it a huge joke, and I managed to get a drink of milk from the garage attendants for her. Really enjoying her novel way of refreshment, we hoped she would not need the bowl for it's real purpose.

On our return to Woolton, there was a patient waiting to go to theatre. Most of the nurses were very keen to go on theatre duty, as I was very intrigued to discover the fascination they had I went too. After wheeling our sleeping patient alongside the operating table, she was transferred by the theatre staff on to the table. Instead of returning to the ward as I should have done, I donned theatre gowns, and remained inside. "Are you staying?" I was asked.

"Yes," I replied.

Standing well back, I did nothing but listen to the casual chatter of the theatre staff. As the surgeon made his first incision, "This is a tough old bird," he remarked. Not the kind of talk I ever dreamt went on in the theatre, and reflected would he have said the same about my appendix had it come to anything. As I stood there watching the blood begin to appear, and the artery forceps being placed in position, I seemed to drift into a world of make-believe. All the nurses, Sister, and the surgeon appeared to be cut out of cardboard. Feeling as though in a trance, I was only conscious of the deep breathing of the patient.

"Are you alright?" filtered through my invisible screen.

"Yes thanks," I replied and wondered at the question, but realised I would be no good as theatre staff. Having returned our patient to the ward with the familiar smell of ether, I took the empty trolley back to the theatre. Returning an empty trolley to theatre is great fun, if two of you happen to be going the same way. Especially if one gets aboard and the other races madly down the long corridors skirting the corners. Until you get caught.

At last there was another New Zealand girl in the hospital.
"I believe you come from New Zealand?" a new patient greeted me with. It was so nice I thought to have someone from my own country, even though she was a Wren, and not in the same section of the Navy as me. When she tried to draw me in to singing Maori action songs, I felt like a fish out of water, as I had long forgotten them, and didn't realise until then how very English I had got even to my speech. Unfortunately after her discharge from hospital, she was transferred to another base.

Being on an early shift, and as reports had come back that the lunch wasn't up to much that day, I rescued a fair meal from what was left on the food-trolley. This we usually did when we wanted to get away early. Hiding it under a towel on the edge of the bath when Sister was busy, we would slip in and swallow it and so get away really early. To dodge Sister that day had us all on hot-bricks. Eventually our opportunity came, two of us slipped in for a hasty lunch. With very bad table-manners, we heard someone coming. Before we had time to hide our sins Sister stood watching us. I think she was taken by as much surprise as we were. For what seemed ages, we stood speechless and thoughtful. Not knowing what to do or say we just felt guilty. Presently a wry smile crept across her pensive face. "Don't get caught will you, and don't pinch mine," she ventured. Happily smiling she left us to swallow the rest of our hasty meal.

Racing off duty and back to the Gables, I hastily changed and left for the Empire Rendezvous. The Kiwis had been waiting and hoping I would show up at the Rendezvous, as they had the news that the Hospital-ship Maunganui was in Glasgow for a refit and I may catch her. Straight away I went to the Quiet Club and wrote to Mr. Jordon again, then went on to a dance with one of the boys.

There was a great crowd at the large dance-hall that Jo took me too with officers and men mixing freely. Many girls in uniform were there, as well as civilians. Some of the girls had such fantastic hair-dos, they reminded me of a bird-of-paradise in hysteria.

Dancing round and swopping partners in a *Paul Jones* with all the light-hearted gaity and teasing that was part of our relaxation, I found myself partnered by a very junior officer whose rather supersilious manner gave me the impression that it was a bit of a blow to find he was dancing with just a V.A.D. Supporting his obvious egotism, he invited me to have a drink. I accepted his offer as I had lost sight of Jo, and anyhow I felt I may as well make the best of my off-duty hours. If I was lucky enough to get on to the Maunganui, nursing conditions would undoubtedly call for greater self-discipline than we had to exercise on land. We would also be more vulnerable on the high seas even though she was well marked as a hospital-ship.

Having handed me a small drink, "I'll bet you nurses have a wonderful time with your patients," he remarked with an undesirable suggestive sneer in his voice.

Revolted I did not know what to say. After a pause, "Yes we do," I told him casually. "A few weeks ago two of us spent most of a whole morning redressing the hideous wounds for a patient who had both his legs amputated. As soon as we had finished our mammoth task, our patient jovially offered to take us to a dance when he got his artificial legs. What's more I intend to accept his invitation, and he is only a rating." I felt I wanted to burst into tears, as there was too much tragedy and self-sacrifice by both officers and men for any smugness. I could do nothing else but hand him his drink back, and suggest he find more adequate company next time.

On the way back to the Gables, Jo who was a varsity student prior to joining up, asked me to go out with him the next day.

70

Individual dates were a pleasure I most declined, for fear of hurting some decent person as life and movements were so uncertain that I did not feel free to allow anything other than just casual friendship to lighten my off-duty hours. If there was ever the remotest suggestion of seriousness I was off.

I had not long before been out a few times with a very decent airman and began to feel very sad when in all earnestness he often remarked "How I wish you were an English girl." Providence took a hand before it became too deep, and he was sent away to the Middle East, giving me a sincere quotation before he left.

Thoughtfully mounting the stairs and going to my room, I wondered who was in my bed, and in my pyjamas? Going over to investigate, I found someone had dressed up a cricket-set, placing it in my bed and completing the job with a tin hat. The next afternoon joining Jo and four other Kiwis, we went to see a wrestling match. I had never seen one before and was revolted by it. For a change we all went to a stage show. One of the items was a cowboy spinning a lasso round and round himself, while he cracked jokes. Fortunately they were so suggestive I couldn't see through them. One was over the limit, but was so clever, that even though I felt embarrassed I couldn't help giggling inwardly. Suddenly a sharp dig in the ribs from Jo's elbow stopped me. Whispering in my ear, "If you were a nice girl, you wouldn't know what that meant."

"If you were a nice boy you'd take me out of here," I whispered back. We all did leave and had a much happier time at the Rendezvous. Unfortunately this was the last time I saw any of them, as they had been posted.

◉

THE CROSSROADS

Shortly a reply came through from Mr. Jordon containing the news it could not be arranged for me to join the Maunganui as they only had authority, to accept new members from New Zealand or the Middle East. For the first time I was almost driven to despair.

Word had come through that all wards had to be cleared as much as possible in readiness for D.Day. It was very difficult to keep ourselves occupied all the time. All the patients that could not be sent home received almost individual attention.

Some of our nurses were being posted overseas. I was hoping that if I could get to the Middle-East, I could then perhaps transfer. Betty had been posted to Simonstown. Lucky Betty. I always remembered her being asked by a doctor to wash his pyjamas. She did. Then stitched his pocket up containing a note: Laundress by appointment.

Passing down the corridor towards the mess-hall for afternoon tea, I couldn't believe my eyes. Crowding the entrance hall, and half way down the corridors, one had to pick one's way stealthily between a maze of stretchers. The sight was appalling. Every nurse remained on duty and worked ceaselessly and untiringly, until every patient was settled comfortably in bed and all his belongings had been recorded in detail. There really was action somewhere and our wards were soon overflowing. Eventually getting off duty, I managed an early night, but was too tired to sleep.

Apple and her companion came in on late passes, unaware of the hectic afternoon we had had, as they had gone ashore before our sudden influx of patients had arrived. Someone with a taste for fun, had apple-pied their beds. Creeping upstairs like a pair of elephants, they soon discovered it. Happy Apple made up her mind, that if she had to make her bed at midnight, so could the others. Amid stifled hilarity they began turfing the others out of bed. As I couldn't sleep and had heard all this I slipped under mine. When they discovered my bed was empty they proceeded to strip it. While they were busy, I gingerly felt round and grabbed a leg. This resulted in a very loud scream to be followed by the head nurse racing upstairs. "Here she comes, get into bed," someone whispered aloud. By the time she had reached our room, it was amazing for her to find us all asleep. After she had left, Apple and her companion had to get out to change.

Time went on and I was soon back on the Wren's ward, one of the nurses had been called home urgently as her mother was seriously ill. A twinge twisted my heart, but with such lovely friends as Jane, Paddy and happy Apple who always raised a laugh when things looked blackest, I had great compensation. Also poor Mary, a friend and I had affectionately nicknamed Big Bertha, when one evening she clumped down the dimly lit corridor, startling us when we were deep in conversation. Had it been Sister the circumstances could have proved rather difficult to justify. With partings so frequent, uncertain and long, to get alone to discuss problems relevent to ourselves, one had to snatch any available time and place, orthodox or otherwise. When two hearts begin to knit in mutual affection, the vast range of problems to face in wartime seem to become innumerable, but still have to be solved. All the Kiwis I had met and become friendly with, whose cheery company meant so much to me, and all my wren patients, and most of all Joy, more than compensated for my isolation.

During my broadcast home I had met Bill, who had arranged for food parcels to be sent to me from the National Patriotic Fund Board in New Zealand. I had also received a very nice airgraph from his wife in Tauranga. This did much to give me more heart. The lovely big fruit cake my mother had sent, was shared by most of my colleagues, as such were rare luxuries in England at that time and brought a touch of joy to us all.

One lunch time after I had only been on the ward for a fortnight, Matron asked me to go off duty, as I was to go on duty on F1 that night. All the S.B.A.s (Sick Berth Attendants) had been sent to handle the casualties, as a result of the landing in France.

Nervously descending the steps to the offender's ward, the position made worse by lack of sleep, I was greeted on arrival at the cabin door "An angel from heaven." Wondering if my chicken's bottom had sprouted wings my nervousness was replaced by an intuition that I would have no need for any worry. Taking over from the day staff, I was advised that one patient was liable to play up, but not to worry as opposite him was an S.P. (Special Police) who, unknown to him, was keeping an eye on him. In the event of any trouble, I was to approach him straight away. Comforted by this information, I felt no different than on any other ward. There were no night treatments, only stomach wash-outs at 5 a.m. The nights passed without incident. Every morning they made a cup of tea for me, and left it on the window-sill for when I could drink it, and every morning, there lined up, were no less than eight cups of tea. I was happy on that ward. The patients themselves did most of the work, leaving me just the night report to write up, and I managed to catch up on all writing and mending.

At breakfast one morning, I was surprised to be told that I was on M11(2) that night.

"But I can't be," I queried aloud, "I've only done a fortnight."

"I'm sure I saw your name on the noticeboard," I was told. Bewildered by this information, I checked the noticeboard and then approached my prospective successor, only to learn she wasn't very well, and as she had heard that I was on an easy ward, had asked to go on it.

Fury flew through my veins. At best she was one of the very few, who found fault with every little thing, and found so many unnecessary complaints about almost everything connected with our temporary, but important way of life. Feeling a suspicion of animosity I contemplated on the position, as I knew Matron would not listen to a petty grievance. To lodge one of this nature could only bring the result it deserved. Putting it aside as just an annoyance I went to bed.

Sleep would not come. Oh boy, if only I were a man I thought, I could punch her on the nose and so satisify my irate feelings. When I was so crook, and had to contend with burning eyes, a high temperature, and the almost unsuppressable longing to give in and have a really good rest, as did many of my colleagues at one time or another, including Sister who once looked like a walking corpse but no one could get her to have just one day off. I was so furious that after a couple of hours of fruitless effort of trying to sleep, I dressed and went ashore. The injustice that persisted made me biff my pillow in disgust, both at how unfair some people could be, and at myself for allowing such a trivial thing to haunt me.

For the rest of that day I tried hard to dismiss it from my mind, and be the obliging nurse some thought I was. Only the thought I had an object in mind kept me from disappearing to Jo's. Soon stupor induced by lack of sleep began to torment me. M11(2) was surgical, and I loved surgical work, and there were many treatments to be done which encouraged me on duty. Penicillin had been introduced and was known as the wonder drug, having saved countless lives from infection of innumerable amputations and horrifying wounds.

I arrived late and all treatments had been done. I was too exhausted for reading or writing. Resting my head on my hands for a few stolen minutes rest I must have dozed. In the far away distance I could vaguely hear Sister coming down the corridor, but I could not move. I felt paralysed. I moved a finger so I knew I was still alive, and it registered I had what we called night-duty paralysis. I could not move as she entered the cabin.

"You know you should stand when I come to do rounds" she thrust at me, followed by a fair blasting.

Slowly in sheer fury, "Blaze away as much as you like!" I thrust back at her. "If you were as tired and disgusted as me, you wouldn't be able to stand either."

"I'll have to report you for this."

"O.K." I shot in. "Do what you like, I don't care any more" struggling it through my aching throat from wanting to burst into tears. Searching in vain for my self-control and respect, I resigned myself to a good pep talk in the morning.

When the day staff came on duty, I was extremely tired, but the verbal explosion in the middle of the night had relieved my feelings. I felt I had just enough energy to cope with breakfast, have a bath if a bathroom was empty, and then sleep it off. This wasn't to be as there was a notice on the notice-board that I had to report to Matron at 9a.m. So the explosion had kicked back. If I was to be dimissed and she blew up too, I only hoped she would blow hard enough for me to land back in dear old Auckland.

Rather apprehensive, but too tired to care, I gently knocked on Matron's door. Nervously I entered her office, responding to her request to do so. As though nothing had happened, she simply asked me what my story was. Listening calming to what I had to say, she quietly answered by saying "You realise Nurse you must be prepared to go any ward you are sent on." Acknowledging this fact, I pointed out it was not the ward, but the unfairness I felt about the whole thing. Appreciating my point too, no more was said, except with a comforting complimentary remark, it would not happen again.

Exhausted and relieved, I made my way to bed and did not move till the evening. Feeling the benefit of a really good sleep, I went on duty forgetting my first landing on the mat. Completing all dressings and treatments, with lights out I emptied the biggest ash-tray I could find, and made my pot of stew for the night. Joy was on night duty, as a runner, so I knew I would have company for a change, if she was not too busy or special-watching. Our stew consisted of quarter filling the tea-pot with tea-leaves, and simply adding more water each time you wanted a drink, which was more a case of occupational therapy. By morning it was so black, one almost needed a pick to get it out of the pot.

P.O.W.s were slowly coming in. They were not in as bad shape as we expected, although they bore visible evidence of physical mis-handling.

Silently doing my rounds, walking past the foot of the beds of sleeping patients with my shaded torch facing the floor, I was startled by a patient suddenly sitting bolt upright in his bed, and yelled, "Where's the bloody dog?"

Stopping immediately "Shh! You'll wake the patients," I whispered.

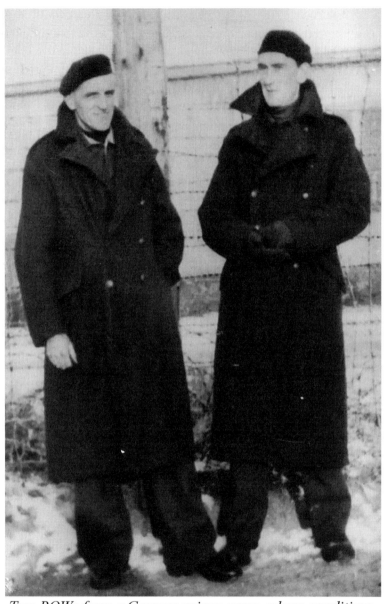

Two POWs from a German prison camp, where conditions weren't as bad as in some

"Oh Nurse it's you: I thought I was back in camp. The guards used to come round in pairs, to pick out who was to be shot next," he whispered.

As I slowly walked up the side of his bed, "You're back in England now, and quite safe. Have a cigarette if you want to and I'll bring you in a cup of tea." I did not give him my stew, and while I was making a fresh pot, I felt a sympathetic lump rise in my throat. His profound appreciation for a simple cup of tea, made me sadder than ever.

"I hope I didn't frighten you Nurse," he whispered as I took it in to him.

"For a moment I wondered what was wrong, I hope you'll be alright now," I answered.

"I'm fine now thanks, and I promise never to frighten you again, even if you do wake us up to see if we are asleep." he chided. "We had a mongrel dog in our camp, and shared all we had with it. Once a Red Cross parcel helped to save its life. When the guards found out, they threatened to bayonet it, if they had, I think we would have all gone beserk." Leaving him in a much happier frame of mind, I returned to my cabin.

A chance remark that disclosed the merest suggestion of the integral part these heroic men had played in concealing the severe mental anguish they had been forced to suffer. Surely their courage and tenacity, coupled with their unfailing sense of humour, was an inspiration to us all. Only these steadfast qualities could now pull them through the heartrending realisation, that they were really free men again.

Joy relieved me last to get my supper, as she was not busy, and was going to remain on my ward until morning. Leaving her with nothing to do, I made my way to the mess-hall. Passing our sittingroom, I was consumed with fear as I saw a ghost at the entrance of our sittingroom. Some of the nurses had mentioned seeing one in white in the grounds, as it was believed there was one. Racing with burning cheeks I alarmed those who were at supper. Staring at my very sudden appearance, no one spoke. Bursting out laughing as I sat down, I realised it was my own reflection on the glass door. It took me some time to live it down, but I looked the other way whenever I passed our sittingroom.

Around two in the morning, the cruelest hour on night-duty for keeping awake, Joy and I had competitions to see who could make the best smoke-rings. With a mountain of butts almost spilling over our giant ash-tray, we were satisfied with our achievements. Turning our art into trying to get them to float round the door, we were startled by a finger appearing in the middle of one of the rings. There standing with a scintilating smile was Sister. "Anything to report?" she asked.

"No, Sister," I replied. Happily she went on her way to complete her rounds of the other wards.

Back on duty the following night, it was a bit of a disappointment to find Joy had a ward of her own, as one of the other nurses had gone to sick bay. My report book showed one patient had not returned from shore leave. Troubled I found he too was a P.O.W. I did not want to report him and hoped Sister would be held up somewhere so that I couldn't.

Luck was in my path. Sister raced through her rounds, as she was pressed for time. As she swept into the cabin she stopped for a moment, "Everything alright Nurse?" she hurriedly asked.

"Yes thanks Sister," I answered just as quickly holding my breath in case my missing patient appeared on the scene. As Sister swiftly rustled back along the corridor after a brief appearance on wards 1 and 111, I breathed a sigh of relief. "Ring F 11 if you need me Nurse, I may not be round again unless you do," she conveyed between my ward and half way down the corridor.

After finishing all dressings and treatments, and getting the lights out, I made my nightly stew, emptied my huge ash-tray, and uneasily settled down hoping my patient would soon show up. If only he would return I would have been much happier, but he didn't. The night passed uneventfully, till doing my two hourly rounds, one patient seemed very restless. I was soon able to settle him again, and also gave him a cup of tea, but not my stew. For some obscure reason he impressed me. He did not pass the usual false flattery that so many of the younger ones did. These I always accepted as a warning, beware a wolf. Nine times out of ten, a date was suggested, and nine times out of ten, on checking a bed-ticket for a single man revealed next-of-kin: *wife.*

Conversation with him, though I did not know him seemed mutual, natural and unguarded. In my cabin that night, for some unknown reason I checked his bed-ticket. Next-of-kin: *mother.* Filled with an unanswerable ponderance, I put it under all the other bed-tickets, but my mind remained impressed. Don't be stupid, you're overtired, I told myself. All was quiet and still. For heaven's sake show up, hung in my brain, as I would almost risk anything rather than report a P.O.W. The silence and stillness was suddenly shattered by a loud tramping down the tiled corridor accompanied by an even louder non-melodious voice. Swiftly going out to stop him, I was met at the cabin-door with a booming "Hello Nurse!" meticulously slurred through the several he had had over the eight.

He proceeded to produce from behind his back, a small miserable, handful of bruised and withered flowers. With amazing alacrity he explained to me that he had spent ten shillings on the best nurse in the hospital, but that was yesterday, and he would get me more tomorrow. The task of matching my five foot light statue against his over six foot heavy one, required an overwhelming amount of tact and persuasion to get him to go to bed. Eventually the task was achieved, and all was peace and quiet again. I understood a drunk person who once hit the pillow, was a very heavy sleeper and I was relieved to return to my cabin. As I was about to rehabilitate myself with my stew, a loud "Nurse!!" bellowed out from the ward. As I walked towards his bed, he held out something to me saying, "Here Nurse have a bite." Investigating his generosity first, I found it was an oversized onion. I threatened to call the S.B.A if he didn't keep quiet, knowing darn well in my own heart he would almost have to wreck the joint before I did so, but my threat worked.

The next morning he asked me what time he got in, and though he did not know what had happened, he did remember buying some flowers for me and wondered if I got them.

Going off duty my mind was again consumed with the ponderance over the patient I had given a cup of tea the night before. It was so silly and unprecedented but very real. I was certain he has a girlfriend, and thought I was just being stupid.

Returning on duty that night, I was compelled to do his dressing first. The hand of providence must have influenced my sudden change of heart, as while entering the ward from the corner of my eye I had a faint suspicion that the patient opposite was not decent. Querying this, "I'm afraid not," came the reply. I know how to handle that I kept to myself. There were many personal duties that sometimes had to be done for our patients, but a flagrant violation of common decency could not be tolerated by either the nurses, or their fellow patients. I continued on, by-passing his bed each time, until all dressings except his were completed. Sister Woof was nightduty Sister. She was always a very bright, lively and efficient person, who could surely blow her top if you were bungling a job. Without hesitation, she would always get stuck into it to straighten things up, and to freely pass on any of her vast knowledge to help you. If the task was a difficult one, she never failed to admit it and would finish it herself. She was a great sport and was very popular with both nurses and patients alike, but had the intellectual capacity to command the rightful respect due to her as a Sister.

I deliberately waited for her in the cabin, continuing to break up and dissolve the large blocks of ship's cocoa for the patient's night drinks. "All dressing done Nurse?" she asked as she entered the cabin.

"No, Sister." Normally I would not admit that unless there was a legitimate reason. Before she had time to come in with anything I told her one patient was indecent.

"Oh I like that kind," she smiled, as she deliberately pushed up both her sleeves and took my dressing tray, and just as deliberately disappeared into the ward. Whatever she said or did I do not know, but I never encountered the same trouble again.

With all dressings and treatments completed, I found myself once again in deep conversation with the patient who had impressed me so much. What was happening to me, I had never in my life been so impressed with anyone. My long heart-breaking efforts to get home seemed unimportant now. I was afraid when I found he had no girlfriend, for I knew if I gave my heart it would be for life, no matter what happened. I did not want to fall for an English boy, I felt it would not be fair, my home, my family, my career. I had so many lovely friends, but somehow they took second place. As time went on, a terrific bewildering transformation had changed my whole outlook. Every day we exchanged letters. As soon as I went off duty, I decided I would not write any more as I finished yet another letter.

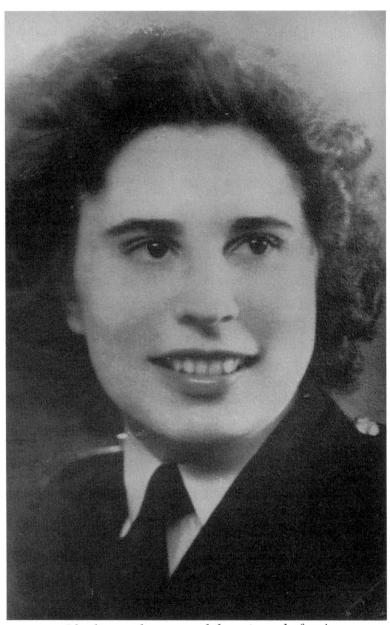

I had never known such happiness before!

I discovered too that his watch had a second hand which was just the thing for taking temperatures. Willingly he lent it to me, but I would borrow it and take only half, return it, and borrow it again later and take the other half, never dreaming how deep our friendship was to become. When he was discharged, he was sent on a gunnery course in Liverpool, which meant we continued our happy friendship and were able to go to shows, pictures, and dances at the Rialto, or for a change to cross in the ferry to New Brighton to the play-ground, and ride on the ferris wheel.

I had never known such happiness before. Neither had the buttons and the insignias on my uniform, or my shoes had so much polishing. When we only had a very short time together, there was always the park quite close to the hospital to saunter in. One evening happily arguing flat out, we forgot the time and got locked in. It was much more fun to scale a brick wall, than to walk through an open gate.

With an invitation to visit his home, I felt very shy, but the affection had grown so strong that I decided to accept. Arriving at his home after a long tiring train journey in the heat of the summer, it was heaven to wash and freshen up. His people's natural sincerity made me feel so much at home and welcome. Once again an English family had shown their generosity and warmth of heart. I knew I could be very happy there. That evening feeling very tired after the long journey and meeting so many new people, it was very relaxing to slip into the comfort of fresh clean sheets over what seemed a very soft mattress. I sank down and just lay back on my pillows. A feeling of peace and calm, made me wonder still more over this sudden change, tempered with something beautiful and new, but I knew nothing till I was awakened by the click of the door-knob to my room the next morning. The whole world seemed at my feet. Nothing seemed to matter, this place was so friendly, so homely, and so unpretentious. The fear this must not get too deep seemed as far away, as did the war and my V.A.D. life. To analyse my feelings only created a mental confusion, or was I sub-consciously concealing the truth. Only one thing was clear, I knew this would never happen again and I would never experience the beauty and radiance of the last few months again.

Up, wash, dress, breakfast and a mad rush to catch my train, put a sudden fullstop to a very happy weekend.

Sitting alone and thoughtful on my bed back at the Gables, reliving all that had happened over the past few months, one of my colleagues enquired after my weekend as was usual. "Yes thanks, I had a much better time than I thought I would, as I was going to a strange place," I smiled to her.

Thoughtfully smiling she asked, "I thought you only went out with New Zealanders?"

"Yes I try so hard to keep to that, but for some unknown reason my veneer has crashed, and I'm getting pretty worried in case I get a chance to get home, even though it doesn't seem so important now," I told her.

When my friend had returned from leave, I forgot all my worries, but both realising how serious the nature of our friendship had developed, gradually many problems began to loom up like a barrier between us, and no matter how we tried we could come to no mutual agreement. Rather than hurt each other each time we tried to come to some agreement I felt it was better not to go out so much and nearly broke both our hearts.

If I decided to marry him I wanted us to be happy for life and not just for a time. My conscience began to bother me, was I being fair? It was obvious that he was very worried too, and was making every effort to do his best for our future. With an overseas draft coming up, we wanted to come to some agreement.

Returning early one evening I sat on the top of the stairs leading to our rooms, suddenly feeling sapped of all energy and enthusiasm. Racing carefree up the stairs one of my colleagues cheerfully remarked, "You're back early Kiwi, have you had a row?"

"No, we just have problems and I would give anything to have them straightened out before he goes to sea."

"If you love him, marry him, remember there's a war on." Slowly I went to my room, she didn't understand either. War is temporary. Marriage is permanent. I had written to my mother hoping she could give me a helping hand, but apart from mail taking months to arrive, it sometimes lay at the bottom of the sea.

So many had given their lives that we may live in peace, and I never dreamt that one single person could come to mean so much to me. I had lots of other friends, with whom I was still in touch by mail. Sadly I wondered had I come to the crossroads, and was really meant to stay in England after all. If only we could come to some agreement, if only I could see my mother for just a short time, I could rest my weary and confused brain. I always thought that when people were in love, they enjoyed an exclusvie happiness all their own, but the real happiness that seemed so near, now seemed to be getting further and further away. In an element of despair and hopelessness, I went to bed to try to sort out my true feelings, and wondered why in these days of so much tension and confusion, had come up against such a situation. If I decided to marry and was left alone with a child I feared that I would not be able to do justice to it.

We had already said good-bye four times, and each time the strain increased. As we said good-bye for the fifth time, I had a strange foreboding that this would be for an unknown time, but could neither understand this fear, or even make mention of it, as I knew how he was feeling to be going on overseas duty. Little realising how true it was to turn out, or how much sorrow there was to follow.

As my tram loomed up through the darkness, I was saddened for the first time in my life by a parting. Whatever happens now, I'll never forget inscribed itself indelibly on my heart.

Selecting a seat in the tram so as to be on my own, its noisy rumbling soon drowned out his footsteps, as he made his way towards his ship. I was so pleased he could not see the tears that now blurred my vision, or know how empty I felt as I was returning to the hospital. Silently I prayed that God would protect him, in the long lonely hours out in the open on the desolate Atlantic Ocean, and bring him safely home again.

The tram seemed to mercilessly crash every rail and sway abnormally tossing an empty heart with it. People talked and chatted quietly amongst themselves, and every stop seemed to jerk me back to earth again until the tram moved off, at the command of the bell, which the conductor automatically tugged, to allow passengers to alight and come aboard.

A soldier came aboard and sprawled his arms across the full length of the seat in front of me. He turned and in a thickened slurry manner through his drink sodden breath, "Hello a nurse," he murmured. "Excuse me nurse you're good girls you are, I'm drunk I know I'm drunk here nurse I'm sorry I'm drunk. Look nurse most o'me mates was killed, but I got out O.K. here take this." Fumbling, slowly and carefully in his drunken stupor, he drew from his breast pocket the most magnificient mother-of-pearl rosary, threaded on a silver chain, I had ever seen. "You take it nurse, a drunken fool like me doesn't deserve them. I got 'em in Italy. You're doing a grand job you 'ave 'em."

Contemplating him and the rosary in serene thought, I wondered what this returned young man had been through.

His eyes though bleary, told of great mental suffering and sadness, but he showed no visible evidence of physical suffering, I felt sure his normal environment was not of this type. Looking back from the exquisite rosary to him, "Please put it back in your pocket," I earnestly asked him.

"Don't you like it, you don't get 'em like it here," he slurred again looking rather hurt.

"Yes I do very much, but you are worthy to have them. Please put them back and treasure them, and don't ever give them away."

"Or right nurse," and it seemed to register that he should keep them. "You know if it wasn't for you girls I wouldn't be here. I'm sorry I'm drunk, if I wasn't I would take you out." Ironical I thought when my own heart was so laden. I sincerely hope that my unknown soldier passenger still has his exquisite rosary.

Without realising I was there, our happy homely Gables appeared in the faint moonlight. Automatically leaving the tram, still lost in my own thoughts, I sauntered back the few yards from the tram stop, passing no-one and almost lifelessly climbed the stairs to my room. Suppressing the urge to flop on my bed and burst into tears, I collected my toilet gear and went to run a bath. Phyl was already nearly through her wash, and with a glistening wet face mumbled through her towel, "Hello Kiwi, you're back early, did you have a good time?"

"Yes thanks," slipped through a smile as I disappeared into the bathroom. How long I stayed there I do not know.

Never again would I race out just in time to catch a tram, finishing polishing my buttons as I went. Knowing and almost taking for granted what I knew would be a very happy afternoon or evening. To return to find some prank played on me, or my freshly ironed clothes hidden, or my bed tampered with, or someone else going through our happy mill of tricks. To forget for a short time my patients, the routine. Work went on as usual no one knowing how heavy my heart still was. Each day hoping he was safe and had not met any U boats. Thinking now he may be somewhere near Ireland. He may be on watch. Many of my colleagues must have felt the same at some time or another, and I felt ashamed I hadn't more courage. After a few days I tried to accept my position and placed my soldier passenger's story before mine.

ON DRAFT

It was a God-send to look forward to another weekend with lovely Joy, as I knew I could have the most pleasant time I could wish for. This time we had to travel by train. Boarding the taxi at the Gables, I offered my share of the fare to Joy. "No Mona, Dad has given me enough for both of us." This touched me very much, as he had already generously given us a wonderful afternoon and evening to celebrate Joy's birthday. We had afternoon tea at the Adelphi in Liverpool, followed by much better seats than we could afford on our Navy pay to see *"This is the Army"*. He had kept this as a surprise for us, but Joy and I could only smile and said nothing, as we had seen it no less than six times. I had been lucky enough to draw a free ticket at the hospital to see the live show and the personal appearance of Irving Berlin. In the evening Joy's father had taken us back to the Adelphi to dine and dance.

The train we travelled in was filled to capacity with service men and women. When we alighted on to the platform in Wales, I felt as though we had entered a foreign land, as everyone was speaking Welsh. Only Joy could understand what they were saying.

Feeling very refreshed after our weekend, we returned to the Gables. A dance was being held in the hospital and we were allowed to bring a partner. I had no partner now and was not going. One afternoon Joy and I had gone to the Empire Rendezvous for a cup of tea, and it was nice to find a Kiwi I knew who joined us. I asked him half-heartedly if he would like to come and bring a partner for Joy. As the Kiwis drifted in he asked them all. I've got a dozen for you Kiwi, and with great enthusiasm they all wanted to come. Explaining I was only allowed one, I agreed to try to get them all in. When the evening arrived I met them all. Bubbling over with mischievousness, we marched up to the main door of the hospital. Showing my pass, I was asked, "Have you got passes for all these?" With this he let us all through. The dance was well under way when we arrived, and the Kiwis were in great demand.

To be dancing and singing to the tunes of *'Pack up your troubles,'* and *'Powder your face with sunshine,'* brought a little sadness to my heart, but I had no time for any real thought, as I was never off the floor. Spotting a weakness of mine, I went over to get some cheese-straws. Standing alongside them was a very unsteady officer, with the oddest interpretation of the English language I had ever heard he addressed me. To try to understand his apathetical affectation would have required all the skill of a student of languages. While I was trying to solve his phonetical effort my partner caught on, and saved the situation by naively balancing a dozen empty beer glasses into his arms. My partner then grabbed me and a handful of cheese-straws and away we went dancing and munching. "If you want any more Kiwi I'll get them for you, he's too drunk to be able to talk." On my partner's return our officer was still standing there nursing his glasses, no doubt wondering how they got there.

'Auld Lang Syne', brought a very happy evening indeed to a close. Joining my dozen partners on the top of the tram returning to the Gables, we had our own special sing song of Maori action songs. Some of us knew the tune, but not the Maori words. This made no difference, as we used Maori place names instead.

Within a few days I was due for leave again. I had almost crossed out the hope of getting home now, so decided to make the best of Kiwi company. Leaving the Gables, I was stopped by the only snob we had. "Take your flashes down," she remonstrated. "It looks ridiculous to have 'City of London' on your shoulder and New Zealand on your sleeve."

"I'll take 'City of London' down but NOT New Zealand " I answered vehemently and stalked away. Booking in at the Y.W.C.A. in Russel Square I went to the New Zealand club for lunch.

HAEREMAI embroidered in huge letters, on a piece of material hung right across the back of the hall, making one feel this was a breath of beautiful New Zealand. Serving lunch was our own lovely talented ballerina Bebe-De-Roland, who at the time was starring in *'The Lilac Domino'*.

When I went upstairs to the writing rooms to write a letter, it brought me right back to memories of home to be introduced to part of our Maori representation of New Zealand's war effort. Our Maori is by nature a thorough gentleman. Commanding by example the great respect of his host country when overseas. I was invited by a New Zealander who lived near Kensington to spend a day with her, and to visit Hampton Court. A beautiful sunny day shone down on us as we explored with great interest the one time palace of King Henry V111. The huge dining table, the wall bath, Queen Victoria's dolls, were all fascinating. Going into the ancient chapel, a service was being held. Penny had thoughtfully brought a rug in case we needed it. As we sat

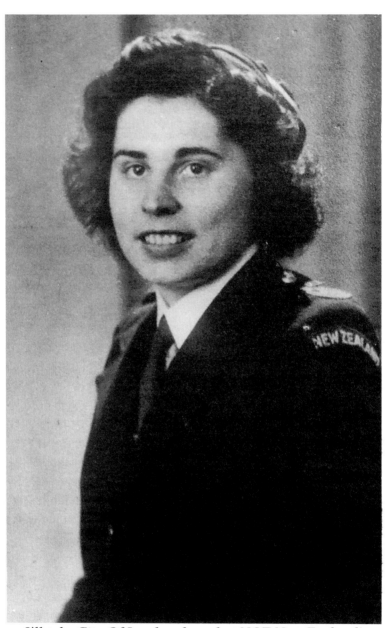

I'll take City Of London down but NOT New Zealand!

at the very back of the chapel, she spread it out over our knees. To our horror she had mistakenly brought her ironing blanket, which was minus an awful lot where the iron had stood too long. She took me to try my sense of direction in the maze. I did very well, and as nearly everyone does, got lost.

There were many ex P.O.W.s at The New Zealand Forces Club in London, and over morning tea, it was suggested that I see Kips as he might be able to help me. Making an appointment for me at his office in Halifax House for the following morning, I duly arrived. Even if he could not help me, it was a great honour to have had the chance of a conversation, with our well loved and respected hero, Sir Howard Kippenberger. Escorting me to the lift, we found it was out of order. Slowing walking and talking down several flights of stairs, it was not until I had spoken of my interview with him, that I learned he had no feet. I arrived back at the club, just after our beloved King and Queen had left. That evening I was invited to share a double complimentary ticket to see Bebe-De-Roland dance in the *'Lilac Domino.'* It was a very beautiful show, and took us away temporarily from the strain of war. Back at the club I was surprised to see Norman, whom I had met several weeks before in Liverpool, but because of his tendencey to seriousness, I did not see much of him. Right or wrong he was going to see me back to the Y.W.C.A. This did not meet with the approval of my temporary escort. Unattached to either I suggested they both see me back. This did not meet with approval either, so I let them sort it out. Much arguing ensued, but when they began to fight it out, I slipped out and went back alone.

The dance the following evening was as spirited as any I had ever been too.

"Hey Kiwi I believe you come from the shaky isles," my very temporary partner teased.

Before I could answer, "Dance with a real New Zealander," said a South Island boy, and so it went on all night.

Leaving fairly early five of them decided to see me on to the tube. Half way there, one of them asked, "Do you want to powder your nose Kiwi?"

"No thanks, she's right, it doesn't matter in the dark," I returned. This answer brought spontaneous mirth from my companions.

"Never mind Kiwi you've got a date at the club tomorrow, and we'll see if we can get a ticket for one of the shows around here."

Glancing at the noticeboard next morning I was puzzled to see a priority telegram addressed to me, stuck behind the tape. Thoughtfully opening it, "Opportunity draft Australia. Wire reply.' came as a bewildered surprise. For a moment I could not believe what I had just read. Immediately I wired back in the affirmative. I was young enough to accept any opportunity that offered to help me to get home. Some of the boys were already at the club as I joined them for a cup of tea. "I'm on my way home boys!" startled them.

"Kiwis can spin a good yarn but that's the best yet," one of them remarked.

"It's true I tell you," I returned calmly.

"This is news boys," they toasted with their cups of tea wishing me a safe journey home. I am sure they did not really believe me, any more than I could belive it myself. "How did you do it?" one enquired.

"Santa Clause!" I answered, adding that I would beat the lot of them. Soon every Kiwi I knew gave me his home address, to visit his people if I did get home first.

"Doc and Rabbit will be disappointed to hear this when they eventually turn up," one of the party told me.

"Never mind, I'll meet them when I get back home," I answered. "Tell them I've gone to powder my nose." Laughing outright cheery good-lucks accompanied my leaving the club, to collect my things from the Y.W.C.A. and return immediately on the first available train to Liverpool.

On the evening of my return, there was a letter waiting for me, in the familiar handwriting I had longed to see. Impatiently I opened it, and then fear gripped me. Would I be here to meet him and explain, or would I too be out somewhere in the mid-Atlantic? Our sailing date was as secret as our destination, and the ship we were to travel on. I knew it lead to the Pacific. The beautiful homely Pacific that surrounded my own country.

England was now sending her sons and daughters out for service in the Pacific. Had it not been for Daphne having married recently, I may not have been one of them.

Kept exceedingly busy with having our passport photographs taken, and passports to be made out, clearances to obtain, tropical kit to purchase, medicals, X-rays, injections, not to mention the great excitement of welcoming and showing our new replacement nurses our routine, I had no time to let my spirits fall. Faced with the problem of making my white dress uniforms, Elizabeth, who prior to the war had been a dressmaker, offered to make them for me. My ward frocks had to be purchased in Manchester. We were each issued with a very large white brazard to wear on our arms in case we were sunk, to signify our status.

"You'll be able to spend your weekends at home now Lassie," a Scotch nurse informed me.

"Not quite," I told her, "but I may be able to spend a leave there."

"Why you're there?" she emphasised.

"I'm afraid that it is a five day journey," I answered her.

"What!" she exclaimed.

"Never mind," I told her, "I'm going to try to get some leave as soon as we get there as it is so much closer to home."

With only two days to go the atmosphere was charged with excitement as nearby relations and friends were visiting the Gables, since we were not allowed shore-leave. The place seemed so crowded with all the new nurses who had arrived to replace those of us who were going overseas. Excitement too was running high for those who were going overseas for the first time in their lives. For me it was an answer to a long struggle, almost too good to be true. "Kiwi - phone!" had to be called very loudly to rise above the excited laughter and chatter. Not knowing who it could be I gayly answered.

"It's not true Mona," came across the line, and momentarily stunned me. Fighting back the tears and overwhelming urge to break ship and go straight to his home, made clarification of thought and stabilisation of emotion almost an impossibility. Not being allowed ashore I could not even meet him half way. He did not have time to get to me, as he had only just arrived back in Glasgow, and rung at his first opportunity. How I kept control is only a miracle. My mind became a blank as I put the receiver down.

Leaving the phone box in a daze, dodging the crowd of happy chattering nurses and relatives in the hall, a sudden scream silenced everyone immediately. Slumped beneath the mail-board was one of our new nurses, who was a most attractive auburn-haired girl, and just come in after an afternoon off, to go straight to the mail-board to collect her mail, as was our practice. Uncontrollably sobbing pitifully, she was clutching almost to shreds a letter that had just bourne the news her husband had been killed. She had only been married three days before. A tragic gloom hung over us all, as even though she had only been with us for such a short time, we all felt her grief.

Wanting to be entirely alone, I went up to bed and disppeared right under my blankets, this time I could not control my tears.

Dismayed and broken, love and life seemed so hard, tumultous and unreasonably hard. I could only think, I've got to see you again, but how and when, but I must go home first now.

It was very hard to hide my very sad heart, and appear to be thrilled to be going home at last, as we all put the finishing touches to our packing. To be leaving behind our happy homely lovely little hospital, that two years before we had so happily prepared for our patients and ourselves. To the mischievous pranks most of us all joined in. The moral and general conduct of all the nurses was to be admired. Their spontaneous and genuine understanding towards one another. Of help, advice, and offers to spend weekends at their own homes, is an honour never to be forgotton. Their sharing of home-cooking, with the severe rationing conditions at the time, reflects the sincere generosity of them all. I would always remember them with pride and gratitude.

J.1

On the 17th. of November 1944 before boarding the Naval transport, which was to take us to Gladstone dock, it was very hard to say good-bye to such a lovely person as Joy. Even on that last day, she had collected my watch from the jewellers and paid for the repairs herself. How I wished she was coming with us.

Sitting silently in the back of the van, for the last time I saw the familiar Woolton tram, and the many places that had been my haunts for so long, as we passed on our way through to Liverpool. On the wharf, standing at the foot of the gangway, dreamily watching our cases being loaded aboard the *'Empress of Scotland'*, an officer approached me and shook hands. Commander Horne from Auckland was on draft too. I had met him once before while making my broadcast home.

Glancing up at the crowds of Naval personnel, that lined the ship's rail, I too made my way up to join them. Slowly the gangway was raised and fastened in position. The great propellors of the troop-ship soon churned the lazy water into a turmoil. Gradually the ship turned. All around me sailors and V.A.D's waved and called good-bye. Sadly gazing back at Liverpool, as it seemed to silently move further away, my heart was left behind. What lies ahead? How long now, before we meet again?

Motionless and alone, "Glad to be going home?" almost frightened me. "Meet Blue, meet Ron," they both said together as two Kiwis stood either side of me. Glad to see them we talked for a while, as England slowly disappeared from sight. Out on the vast open sea, we settled down to ship-board life.

After tea, I went below feeling very tired. Settling into my bottom bunk, I did not know I was to remain there for a few days. The movement of the ship was so incessant. The strong smell of salt water was so nauseating. I felt almost as if I wasn't there. The shock of having a blanket-bath a few days later forced me up on deck. Once there Blue and Ron, again one on either side of me made me walk for miles around the deck. That night I was almost driven to tears with extremely painful leg-muscles. Everywhere we went the decks were dotted with moving sailors. The graceful ship that was carrying me on my first leg home.

As my spirits gradually bucked up, I made up my mind to do something I had always wanted to do. Just travel and learn to know the ways of foreign peoples. Marriage perhaps one day, but not for many many years until I had satisfied my roving nature. The thoughts at this stage brought one fear I hated. Being tied with reponsibilities, until any children there might have been, were old enough to stand on their own feet. The only alternative was to marry a rich adventuresome man, who of course only lives in one's imaginative mind. So it was finish my war service, and prepare for work and study, which I was very eager to get started on as soon as the war was over. I had travelled extensively throughout England, and lived in the Shakespearian country, absorbed the beauty of Anglesey, and seen the gaunt barreness of the mountains round Bangor. Spent many hours visiting the colleges at Oxford, aware of the years of hard solid swot and study of the students that turned out to be so many of our highly learned scholars today. Some of whom I had nursed as patients, and worked with on the B.B.C. Enjoyed the peace and quiet of Buckinghamshire, and watched the boat-race on Henley-on-Thames. Got completely lost in the whirl of London, relaxing on the steps of St. Pauls, and fed the pigeons, in Trafalgar Square.

It was all over now, I had fallen in love, which I had tried so hard not to do, as circumstances and an adventurous nature, could not allow it's beauty to bloom. So with a broken, though in a way a satisfied heart, full of the kindness and hospitality that had made my enforced separation from my family a really happy one, I looked back for the last time, in the direction of England, what had long disappeared from sight, and saw only a blank horizon. Lost in thought I was soon brought back to earth, when Blue and Ron, introduced me to no less than thirty other Kiwis who were travelling on the same ship.

Late one night, while we were preparing to go to bed, the ship gave a mighty jolt, and began to roll insanely from side to side. Startled, in the two berth cabin that eight of us shared, we apprehensively looked across from one to the other, with no-one so much as parting their lips. Peg was already in her bunk reading, and glanced up at Val, who was sitting on her upper bunk casually swinging her legs, making us all giggle like overgrown schoolgirls with her crazy wisecracks. Suddenly as though to keep her balance, she gripped the backs of her knees on to the side of her bunk. Her eyes steadily held mine, as though we were transfixed. Another sudden muffled thud transformed us into breathing statues.

We're in trouble, I dared not to voice, while the butterflies in my stomach made me feel sick. Gradually as the lonely ship away out in mid-ocean settled down to it's rocking and rolling movement, I slowly and gently followed the silent movement of the other girls, and lay my head on my pillow. Those of us who had not yet changed, remained fully clothed. Silently and tensely I closed my eyes. Uneasily I slept for only a few hours, until I went on deck in the early hours of the morning. All seemed in order, the ship was now as steady as a rock. Sleepily others began to gather on the decks, and then rumours flew round the ship, that U boats had been detected and we'd had to zig-zag to dodge them. We had no escort, as they had left us on our own, once we had cleared the coasts of England and Ireland, but our gallant ship with two thousand troupes, and only thirty-two nurses continued on to reach Panama on my birthday.

I was given a New Zealand halfpenny by one of the Kiwis. Something I hadn't seen for almost eight years, and one of the most magnificent butterflies that I had ever seen, that was foolish enough to flit within range of the ship's rail. From somewhere Ron had acquired a miniature hand of very green bananas. We were not allowed ashore, so spent most of our time carving our names on the ship's rail.

Once we had passed from the Atlantic Ocean and through the Panama Canal, an almight deafening cheer went up from all the Kiwis, as she gracefully slipped into the beautiful blue waters of the Pacific Ocean. That same evening gathered aft of the ship, we celebrated by singing Maori songs, which I was picking up all over again. Standing out so clearly in the heavens above, we cheered with excited confidence the sight of our glittering Southern Cross. Only then I think, could I fully comprehend the fact that I was truly heading toward home at last. It was lovely to see the Southern Cross and be in Pacific waters again.

During the day, time was taken up with life-boat drill, which would sound at the most unexpected times. Everywhere we went we had to carry our life-jackets. We were briefed on what to do in an attack, and were told which life-boats to make for if we were sunk.

Our practise smoke-screens were most effective, but with God's guiding hand, we were never required to use them for protective purposes.

One afternoon I was being instructed how to roll a cigarette sitting on the deck in a fair breeze. Blue was a keen sportsman, and had gone to take part in a boxing-match. On his return, looking very much worse for the rounds he had taken part in, he joined us. It was so hot down below, that we decided to have a sing-song on deck that evening. Blue brought his wife's photo up to show me. He wanted me to visit her if I managed to make Auckland, as he was being redrafted from Sydney and would not be able to. Early the following morning, as I was walking round the deck, I saw it still lying where we had been gathered the night before. Although damp from being left out in the open he was very relieved to get it, as he had spent ages searching the overcrowded quarters he had looking for it. I did meet his wife in Auckland and had the pleasure of taking her to my own home for tea, and we became good friends.

With very strict blackout regulations, it became very hot indeed in the crowded cabins and smoke-rooms Struggling through three sets of blackout-curtains on to the deck for a breather, for a time became a respite I could not enjoy, unless I was with the Kiwis. For some unknown reason I was mercilously persued by a creep. There was no other word to describe him. I was not the only one faced with this problem, but was fortunate in having a trustworthy bodyguard.

For a time, Jane, who was with me in Woolton and who had looked after me when I should have been in sick-bay, and myself would sit by the hour, on our life-jackets in the toilet for some peace to talk alone. It was surprising how much we enjoyed our privacy.

One afternoon, even though I was with the Kiwis, my unwanted admirer hung around till he almost gave me the creeps. I mentioned it to my cobbers, and glancing round one remarked, "I don't blame you Kiwi." Not knowing how to overcome this difficulty, one advised me to let him date me and assured me that I would come to no harm.

Immediately I was on my own he pestered me again, so I did as I was advised, knowing I was in safe hands. Duly the appointed time arrived. As I approached the appointed place, alone, he disappeared as all my Kiwi companions stepped forward at the right moment, and I was never bothered again.

Although we had had a safe journey, and most of us had enjoyed ourselves as well as we could, I do not think any of us were sorry to soon be on dry land.

A dance was organised one afternoon, and with cheerful spirits the band gave 'In the Mood' all the pep and speed it could. It took all the energy and breath you had to keep up the pace. The floor was so crowded, and the sea so choppy, that as the ship lurched from side to side, so did all the dancers. An excuse me, gave one only one turn, and then a new partner. Many were unable to get on the floor at all, but lined the windows in merry mood, with jocular remarks adding to the merriment.

With only the Tasman to cross now I felt sick with excitement to see Three Kings disappear behind us, as we passed the northern tip of New Zealand. How I wished we were calling into Auckland.

It seemed almost like fairyland to glide smoothly into Sydney Harbour, and see all the beautiful lights at night, after having spent so many years under blackout restrictions. 'Did you protex yourself this morning' raised quite a bit of mirth, as it shone out in neon lights, clearly visible from where we were anchored, offshore.

Standing on deck the following morning, it was a very pleasant surprise to be handed a telegram of birthday greetings, and 'hope to see you soon' from my family. The ship became a hive of industry as all our cases were unloaded, for an unknown destination. All V.A.D.s boarded waiting buses also for an unknown destination. Settling in the bus, and gazing from the window, it was a very comforting feeling, to know at last I was in my neighbour's paddock, with only thirteen hundred miles to go instead of thirteen thousand. A few hours, in a plane, a few days by boat.

LUCKY SEVENTH

We seemed to travel for hours, disappearing into vast open country, accompanied by heat, which grew hotter and hotter as the atmosphere became dustier and dustier. Nothing but blue-gums seemed to grow everywhere. Civilisation appeared to be left behind. Arriving at a bush camp at Ingleburn, some of us were shown to long wooden dormitories, while others had small wooden huts. Stepping into the heat and dust, the wide cracks in the parched earth, told of drought conditions. The Australians in their slouch-hats all looked very sunburnt and tired.

There was no sleep for us the first night as we were continuously dive-bombed by mosquitoes. Away in the distance, we could see the fierce glow of bush fires. We spent most of our time continously washing our white uniforms. The Australian nurses were one up on us in their smart khaki ones. They were most helpful, and very friendly. Immediately we had acquired some semblance of organisation, and I had not been permitted to remain on the troop-ship we had travelled in, as she was leaving for Auckland, I applied for home leave. Twenty eight days was granted to me from my date of travelling. To get transport home was not an easy task, even from Australia, and took me almost a month to procure.

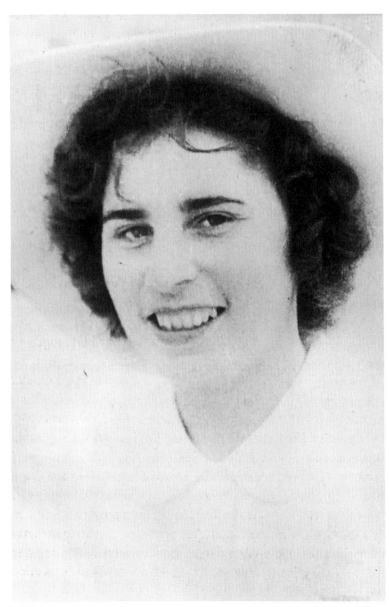

We spent most of our time continuously washing our white uniforms.

Having arrived in Sydney a couple of days before Xmas, and landed away out at Ingleburn in complete isolation except for the barracks of Australian soldiers, nurses, flies, mosquitos, dust, and distant bush-fires, Jane and I enquired if it were possible for us to go to church on Xmas Day. A couple of Australian soldiers offered to take us for a drive to the church. I sat in the back of a small van, while Jane landed a seat by the driver. Just as we were about to leave, Madam came over to enquire as to where we were going. Unknown to me, Jane had said exactly the same as me. "We are going to church Madam." Not looking very happy about it, she reminded us that we were to attend a meeting that night. We couldn't really blame her, if she thought we were having her on. After a very pleasant drive, we arrived at a dear little wooden country church, which seemed so isolated and surrounded by bush. We were back in time for our meeting.

Some of us were invited by the Australian nurses to join them in carol singing on Xmas Eve. After gathering together, we boarded the backs of lorries, each carrying a lantern that had been given to us, and sang all the way as we bounced towards the Officer's mess. This was very novel indeed, and so vastly different from the very impressive Christmas Eve I had spent at Woolton only the year before. We finished the evening with a toast in the Officer's mess.

On my first opportunity I went to Sydney to see about some means of getting home. Making first for the New Zealand club, I had the very great privilege of meeting Nana and Van, who though advancing in years, never failed to turn up to serve tea at the club. I soon found that I had two very lovely friends, and two very lovely homes to spend my weekends, when I was off duty.

Being advised to see Colonel Mothes, who was at the time the New Zealand Liason Officer in Sydney, I went straight to his office. Passing through the Sydney Streets, it was like a land of luxury, as there seemed so much one could buy. His offers to help me were very encouraging. After going backwards and forwards several times to see him, he eventually was able to get me a lift on an airforce plane leaving for Auckland the following morning.

Back at Ingleburn I washed all my uniforms ready to go home. Hanging them up to dry, the burning sun relentlessly stung your flesh, and its glare was blinding. The heat was so intense, unrelenting and exhausting. We all felt it very much, and spent most of our time with as little on as possible. One always felt exhausted and lethargic.

Arriving next morning excited to board the plane, I was told it had crashed on take-off. The following morning a V.I.P. had to be flown over. A third time a Kiwi was flown home on compassionate leave, and there was to be no more planes for some days. Shipping was out of the question, my only hope was Teal (Tasman Empire Airways Limited). Enquiring at their offices, I was advised it would cost around £30 and I had to take my chance on a seat. Reluctantly I had to notify my family and was wondering if I was going to have England trouble all over again.

Returning to Ingleburn, in a not too happy frame of mind, Jane and I walked that evening to a small country cafe. The smell of cooking steak was exceedingly appetising. Going in we were amazed to see real eggs (not in powder form) served with it. Sacrificing most of our pay we hoed in.

Within a few days, my family had written to tell me to get home any way I could, as they had already submitted the money for my fare in Auckland. The next day I went again to Teal, and they advised me they would notify me if a seat became available.

One morning we were asked to practice marching with the Australian nurses. It was so impossibly hot, that Jane and I stood on the backs of the toilets, the only place we could keep out of sight, and watched the others swelter in the heat. Another afternoon when some of our nurses had returned from a day in Sydney sight-seeing, they had brought mangoes back with them. Discovering they did not like them, I had a very wonderful time being a most obliging garbage-can for them.

The cooks commanded my sympathy, as working in very adverse conditions the cook-house was almost black with flies. Having lunch one afternoon, I was wondering if the heat had not affected me so soon, when the meat on my plate began to move. Uneasily tingling with suspicion I carefully inspected it, and just as carefully let it walk. I asked for it to be changed, and one of the nurses dumbfounded me by remarking, "It's only your imagination." Senior or no senior I proved my point reminding her I was now in my own part of the world, and nothing could prevent such occurrences so far out in the bush. Had she not seen for herself, how the flies even landed on your fork while in actual use. My proof was so positive with the evidence to back it up, her own lunch was not touched, and she disappeared in a hurry, with a surprised and revolted expression.

At last I had a seat and was asked to report at 6 a.m. in the morning at the Flying boat base in Rose Bay. After spending the night in the Wentworth Hotel, a taxi called for me the next morning and took me to the next leg of my journey home. After waiting in suspense for my seat number, I was told I would have to return next morning as my seat had to be taken by a priority passenger. I was shocked and disappointed beyond words, as the flying-boat became airbourne. I had to watch it go home without me on board. Immediately I had to wire my family, as they would be waiting for me to alight when it arrived in Auckland.

Livid with rage I stormed back to the club. One of the Kiwis I had met on the ship was there, and had the misfortune to collect both ears full of my fruitless efforts to get home. The impact back-fired with "Blow hell out of them, if they turn you down again Kiwi. You're a darn sight more entitled than half of them for a seat I'll bet."

Nana was also at the club, and made me spend the night with her and would see that I was at Rose Bay on time the next morning. Once again there was no seat. Unaccustomed as I was to forceful, verbal expression, I intently walked up to the counter, and let fly in no uncertain terms demanding a seat on that plane. Smugly efficient, the young desk clerk was insufferably rude. To a young woman who hadn't seen her family for so long, all my pent up emotion and longing to see them unexpectedly released itself in a most unladylike manner, leaving the clerk uncomfortably red-faced. As I returned to my seat to see what would happen, a rather pleasant looking man, left a group of people he was speaking to and went over to the clerk. Before he had rejoined the group of people he had just left, my name and seat number was called. My seventh try was lucky, even if I did have to blow my top to get it.

Boarding the Sutherland Flying boat, was a new experience, as I had never flown before. As the pilot called out "Fasten all seat belts!" the plane revved for take-off. As it became air-bourne I looked out of the window. It struck rather a sad note when I saw a child's boat modelled to perfection had floated out to sea. Pensive I smiled to myself. How dumb can you be. It was a real boat, and being air-bourne, we were gaining height all the time. Comfortably settling in my seat, able to relax at last, the constant drone of the engines, coupled with the slight motion of the plane, made me feel very drowsy. Wrapped in my own thoughts high up over the Tasman, I peacefully pondered what it would really be like to see my family again. All the news from home had been such a joy to read during my long absence from my family. The glaring black

CENSORED stamp right across and almost obliterating the age old date-stamp on the letters that had been my only link with home for so long, often told me news would be old, but was still very pleasing to read. Now after so many years I felt I was almost a stranger, and wondered how we would react to one another. Could I at long last get a transfer to a hospital-ship, and so be able to see them more often. Soon everything began to spin round and round in my brain, and a multiplicity of questioning thoughts flooded in. My excitement mingled with sadness heightened as One Tree Hill caught my eye beneath us.

As we circled preparing to land, the magnificent varying shades of green. The orderly windbreaks that separated the miniature, precisely neat paddocks next caught my eye and lay like a fairyland below us. The clear-cut coastline edged in pure white foam, the seemingly motionless streams and rivers and the once familiar one-storied wooden farmhouses dotted here and there, and the striking beauty of Rangitoto Island which appeared to be such a vivid green, unfortunately gave way to my reaching for a bag for the first time. As we gradually lost height towards Mechanic's Bay, I suddenly felt all in. Our view was completely obliterated by the salty surf splashing on our windows as our plane taxied towards the floating dock. Stepping from the plane on to the pontoon bridge, as I approached the end a stranger stepped forward and asked if I was Miss Plane. Astonished, I answered "Yes".

"Stand there I want your photo," he said.

"Good heavens whatever for?" I enquired.

"I'm from the Press," he returned. Perplexed I let him have his way, but at long last I was with my own family again.

NEW ZEALAND FURLOUGH

I do not know who did most talking, but I was conscious of a lump in my throat. Everyone seemed so happy, and my brothers and sister had grown so much. Mum and Dad did not look so different. Biscuits and cake for afternoon tea, and fine pretty cups with saucers to match, instead of mugs or heavy thick crockery, gave me a feeling of being in a dream world. Ham and salad that was served over a clean white tablecloth, instead of meat with maggots, on tin plates, and long wooden benches to sit on, was worth coming home to. The pleasure of gathering in the comfort of our own sitting-room after tea was really home. The summer heat in New Zealand was so temperate, from that of Australia.

A knock on the door, brought a temporary lull to our continous conversations. Not knowing anyone in New Zealand I was puzzled when my father introduced someone to see me. She was a reporter from the Auckland News, and wanted a story. I felt I could not disappoint her, but as I was still a member of one of the forces, it was not an easy task to give her a non-commital interview.

Next morning a photo and a write up appeared in the Herald. The following week, almost half a page appeared in the Auckland Weekly News. Auckland was certainly showing its appreciation to its service personnel. The beautiful flowers, that Mum had in every room, were all from her lovely garden, together with an abundance of extras given by her neighbours.

That night it seemed almost strange to share a room with my sister again. The bed-wire was made of slats, as since my family had returned to New Zealand in 1941, wire woves were unprocurable. This made no difference to a good night's sleep. I was home.

Next morning it seemed almost odd, to have younger children round you, instead of nurses, and a mother to talk to, instead of your own routine thoughts for the next day's work. I left early and went straight to Red Cross Headquarters in Custom's Street. The welcome was warm and sincere from the Advisory Director. Immediately I was very taken with this very wonderful person, and we were to become lifelong friends.

A long informal friendly discussion ended with her promising to do all she could to help me to obtain my transfer. Following morning tea, after having been introduced to the other members of the staff, I was asked to address a meeting of Red Cross Officers the following week. Leaving the building, I wandered around Queen Street and was amazed at how much one could buy in New Zealand. Turning from Milne and Choyce's window, a man whose face was familiar but I did not know him, smiled hello. I did not even answer. "I was very pleased to see you stick up for yourself yesterday," he told me.

Still blank I questioned, "What for?"

"At the flying boat base," he answered.

"How did you know?" I enquired.

"I gave you my seat," he answered.

"Oh I didn't mean anyone to do that," I told him.

"It's alright, I cross the Tasman on business every fortnight," he replied, and saw me on to my tram.

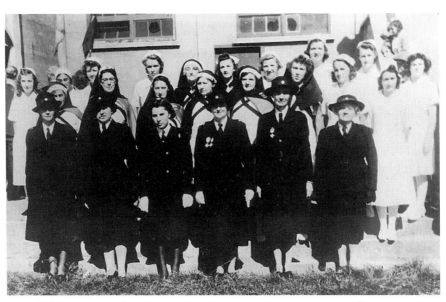

With a gathering of New Zealand Red Cross members in Eden Park.

As mothers will and have a right to, Mum wanted to take me to visit all her friends. A quiet social life, was such a relaxing change, that it was very enjoyable. A trip away out to Massey-Birdwood to visit a lifelong friend was almost thrilling. She had hardly changed in the eleven years since I had seen her last. She was working in her flower-garden when we arrived. As we all talked we walked between the rows and rows of violets and gladioli, picking and handing me an almost perfect bloom, she remarked, "This one is called Miss New Zealand, you deserve it." Her sincerity portrayed to me an appreciation of what our service-men and women were doing. A simple phrase of encouragement to carry in my heart, that our long hours, hard work, and heartbreaks were still well worth it.

I spent as much as I could visiting the relations and friends of all the addresses I had given to me from Kiwis serving overseas. I found this brought great happiness to all I visited.

Soon the morning arrived for me to give my address. To be asked to address a meeting of Red Cross officers, was somewhat of a nervous strain, but to be honoured with such a privilege, gave rise to deep thought, to justify the trust they placed in me. I felt I had to be a worthy representative not only for the Royal Naval V.A.D.s who were my colleagues, but also as a New Zealander. I spoke factually and simply, as they only wanted the truth. I spoke of how their own relatives were faring overseas, and felt it an excellent opportunity to express the sincere appreciation of the many Kiwis I had met, whose morale was kept high, by their unceasing efforts at home, to keep the Red Cross parcels and comforts going. I told of how much joy my own parcel had brought not only to me, but also to my colleagues at Woolton.

Their appreciation and remarks proved my address had been a success. This gave way to more requests to address gatherings further afield and for other organisations too. Making my way to catch a tram, I felt highly embarrased when a stranger came up to me, and said "Hello Miss Plane, I'm so glad to meet you." I was rather glad when my tram pulled up.

As I boarded it, the conductor very cheerfully remarked, "How do you do Miss Plane," and refused my fare.

This was awful I thought on my way home. Making straight for my bedroom to take off my uniform, I gasped as I approached the mirror. I had forgotten to take off the large white disc with my name and guest speaker written on it.

Feeling the benefit of my change, with all my social calls completed to the friends and relations of the Kiwis overseas, I wanted to do something to fill in time while awaiting my transfer. Dad suggested helping him in his office. This really appealed, as I could get my hand in again on the typewriter.

To my great delight a few days later, there was a letter at home for me from overseas. It had followed me half way round the world, and gave me great relief to realise that partings and heartache were only transitory if your heart was true. My whole world seemed to light up again. With so many British ships coming to the Pacific I was hoping for that chance to see him again, so that we could straighten out our problems, now that I had been home and able to see my people.

Calling in at Red Cross Headquarters periodically to see if any news had come through, it came as a severe blow that I could not transfer. Undaunted, a further effort was made for me to be released so that I could join the New Zealand forces. With this hope in mind I was advised to study for an exam in hygiene as this course was necessary to qualify as a V.A.D. in New Zealand. I would then be ready should my release come through. Pending further word from the Navy, Mrs. North the Advisory Director gave me the textbook, and when I thought I had mastered it, she would arrange for my exam.

My mother decided that I should have a holiday, and so with my youngest brother we had decided to go to Maraetai for a weeks break. As the bus passed through Howick, so countrified, and yet so close to Auckland, and on to Maraetai I was very taken with the small groups of Maori children who gathered just to wave happily to the passing bus. Dressed in anything from their fathers' old worn-out singlet, to the smartest fairytale dresses I hadn't seen for so long, their innocent little brown faces revealed their gay little natures. Joy and gratitude again filled my heart, to be in the country and atmosphere I loved, and to live once again with the people who were part of me.

Fired with the enthusiasm of at last preparing to go on a hospital-ship, I took my book with me and spent most of my time everyday lying face down to shield my book from the sun, and studied completely hidden by the tall rank grass. Relaxation came from odd half-hours, of lounging and alternately swimming in the warm clear inviting Pacific Ocean that gently lapped the coastline. Like anything worth having, it was difficult to get and I had to work hard for it.

Before our week was up, a telegram arrived asking me to address a gathering in Unity-Hall. Returning alone, I prepared my speech, and made my way in the evening to the hall. Approaching the hall, I lost my nerve when I saw a very large placard outside. 'Guest speaker Miss Plane R.N.V.A.D.' Turning on my heel I went straight to a milk-bar and had a milk-shake. Had it not been for a kindly member, who had recognised my uniform, and who was on her way to hear me speak, I do not know what would have happened. Their understanding, and genuine interest, soon put me at ease, and I was able to honour my privilege.

It proved a very successful address, and the discussions after were most enjoyable. After three hours in the hall, I left with an overwhelming feeling of pride, as I carried an enormous sheath of the loveliest flowers I had ever seen, that had been presented to me. It symbolised something that would live in my heart for all time, as an indication of their appreciation for those of us who were on overseas duty.

When I thought I was ready for my exam I notified Mrs. North and she arranged for it to take place. The night before it was to be held, I relaxed with a Readers Digest. In it was a very interesting article on quartz glass. I read it to a point of studying it. The following day left in a room on my own, at Red Cross Headquarters, I duly answered the questions on my written paper. Successfully answering later my oral exam, it was concluded with, "Do you know anything about quartz glass and its uses?" Repeating almost all I had read the night before, I surprised my examiner but did not tell her how I came to know so much about it. This stroke of luck earned my exam to have been passed with honours.

With this great news behind me, I returned home to freshen up as I had been invited by the Glen Eden Red Cross to judge both a flower show and a cake competition. I reflected on how some of the English boys had tried to convince me that flowers in New Zealand have no scent. I had to take a tram to Auckland and then change. Immediately the tram I had just alighted from moved off I began to cross the street. "No jaywalking allowed" hit my eardrums. Never having heard the expression before, I asked the policeman what he meant. I could not hope to imagine who looked the more surprised. Given a good pep-talk, I walked the extra couple of yards to the pedestrian crossing and made sure there was no policeman around the next time I jaywalked.

Judging the cake competition proved rather a puzzle as such things had long since been forced from the British diet, due to the acute shortages of butter and sugar. The flower-show was even worse, as the outstandingly beautiful displays, more than did credit to the fascinating art of floriculture, both native and imported. I was almost overcome when I was asked to sign autographs, and was again presented with the winning bouquet of flowers.

A further request had come in for me to address yet another meeting. As our holiday had been cut short, all my family had decided to spend a day on Waiheke Island, as the trip there and back was beautiful. Leaving early in the morning, I was being trained to be a real New Zealander all over again, and lay on the sand in the hot sun along with them all. They all took it in their stride, but I was so severely sunburnt, that to put on my full uniform was agony. Never again would I try to acclimatise myself in such a short time to sunbathing.

It was a great thrill to accept an invitation to spend a weekend with some friends in Taumaranui. The car trip around Wanganui on the Sunday afternoon, took us through some of New Zealand's most beautiful bush. The punga ferns and the nikau palms added grace to its originality. The mighty Wanganui river hides in the bush that lines its banks, the annual nesting place of the rare Kotuku, New Zealand's graceful pure white heron. The natural beauty of some of the Maori children we passed had to be seen to be believed. The picturesque Maori Pas, made exclusive by the amazing individual skillful Maori carvings, and even more realistic by the artistic handling of paua shell, giving New Zealand its own treasured culture. The peace and scenic beauty of this lovely place, was in such vast contrast, to flying over and looking down on the magnificent grandeur of the snow-capped Southern Alps.

Time was dragging on, and I was still no further ahead, although I had no need to worry, I wanted to earn my board, so applied for a casual job as a telephonist, but was not accepted as officially I was still a member of the Royal Navy. This was fine I thought, but could do nothing about it.

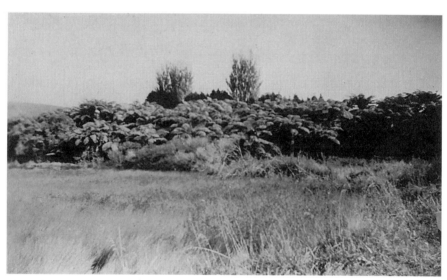

The grace of the punga, taken on a trip round Taurmaranui.

I had made a few friends and we had decided to go to a Maori concert at the Town hall. This was the joy of all joys. To watch again the outstanding skill of the stick-dance, was far too short. The poi-dances were so graceful, and the stocky, strong and powerful build of the men, added character and real lively spirit to the ever popular stirring hakas. Their constant, thundering rhythmic stamping, aroused a vigorous enthusiastic state of controlled excitement. After the show a friend and I decided to round off this outstanding evening with a trip to the small lunapark off Queen Street. Shortly after the *Big Spider* had begun to turn and spin, so did my head and stomach. When it stopped I didn't, and my friend had to help me on to the tram. The journey home only added insult to injury, and he didn't dare come in, so left me at my gate at my request. Mum was rather concerned at the ghost that walked in, but I did not tell her where we had been, as I did not think she would approve of my spinning round being sick high over Auckland.

At last word came through, but not of the best. The Navy would not authorise my release at this later date, and the whole question was being referred to the Admiralty for decision. All I could do was still wait. Another whole month went by, and then word came through that I was to remain on leave until they made a final decision about my disposal. This made me feel a bit like an abstract article. More correspondence, more writing, and I could not take civil employment.

MAY V.E. DAY. Everyone went mad. Everywhere cars, horns hooters, sirens and anything noisy created an uproar. A social life was a relaxing change, but I wanted to finish my war-service out, so went to Red Cross Headquarters again to see if there was anything I could do. With the war over in Europe, a new light was thrown on the possibilities of my remaining in New Zealand, as all efforts would now be concentrated in the Pacific.

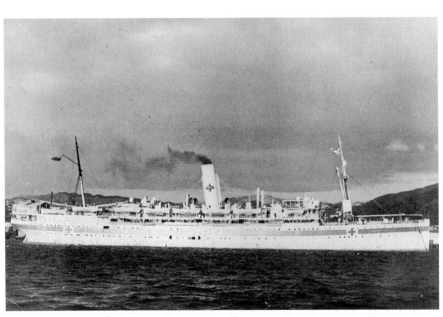

H.M.N.Z. Hospital Ship 'Maunganui'

When the Hospital-ship Maunganui next berthed in Wellington, we took a chance and my name was put on the duty list, and my berth arranged pending Admiralty's decision. A great thrill of excitement went through me. What wonderful news. Excitedly I thought of the thrill of nursing patients in bunks on a rough sea. Where would we go, and how much longer did I still have to wait to achieve my wish. The wait seemed endless.

Speaking at the R.S.A. in Remuera that afternoon gave me a great thrill as I really felt that all my waiting had not been in vain.

Finally word came through for me to call at Red Cross Headquarters. Flying up the stairs two at a time, I was all keyed up to assemble my new kit, and to take orders for hosiptal-ship duty.

The answer when it came was stunning in its impact, as Mrs. North told me the Navy would not release me and that I had to return to Sydney on the first available boat. Feeling desolate and empty, and devoid of enthusiasm, I could find no words to express my thanks to Mrs. North for all the genuine efforts she had made on my behalf, to help me to get my wish. I think she knew just how I felt, as her kind understanding, and good council gave me the courage I needed to accept my position. Thoughtfully I left her office, and made my way slowly back down the stairs and out into the street to board a tram back home.

Perhaps I had expected too much. War was war, and the Navy was the Navy, and I was still part of it.

Mum was very disappointed, and neither of us were very happy at all as I prepared to return to Sydney, as I had to expect that I would probably only get a few hours notice before I had to board ship, and so return to duty.

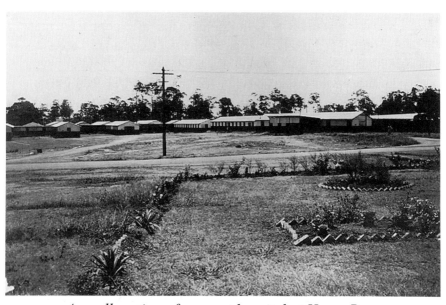

A small section of our vast hospital at Herne Bay.

RETURN TO DUTY

I returned to Australia on a White Star Liner, and was met at the wharf by a naval transport, and taken together with a new surgeon to the Royal Naval Hospital in Herne Bay. All the V.A.D.s who were at Ingleburn temporarily had now well settled in. Arriving at the hospital our Commandant did not seem too pleased when she told me I had to report to Matron's office. Who could really blame her. Six months was a rather long twenty-eight days. As soon as I had dumped my gear I went to find Jane. When I walked into her cabin, she just stared. She thought she had seen a ghost. Rumour had got round, I was having such a wonderful time in New Zealand, I didn't want to come back. In a way she was right, but when she knew the reason and the facts, she was dumbfounded. Instead of going straight to Matron's office I had tea with Jane, and the pair of us simply talked and talked. I gained the impression Matron would not be too hard, and life at Herne Bay was going to be very happy. Many many new nurses filled the V.A.D. quarters as seven other drafts had arrived while I had been away.

Feeling a bit like a fish out of water, I seemed to walk for miles along wooden ramps till I came to Matron's office.

Nervously knocking on her door, she asked me to come in. Greeting me with a very pleasant good afternoon, we only talked of the reason for my long absence, and she welcomed me as she would a new member to her staff. Leaving her office, I thought how naturally charming she was, and wondered whether she realised deep down, what a blow I had suffered.

The hostpital seemed so vast in comparison to our lovely homely little hospital at Woolton. Our quarters spread over such a large area, and our rec-room was so huge, and not the cosy lovely sitting-room we had at the Gables. The whole hospital was eleven miles in circumference.

It was exhilarating to be back on duty. After only a couple of days I was transferred on to night-duty. This could mean anything. I could either get quite a lot of sleep, unofficially of course, if the nurses of the three wards I was runner for didn't need an extra hand, or I could be busier than they, assisting with various duties or special watching.

Reporting to each nurse in turn, I found I had to watch a d.c.l. who had been given approximately only two more hours. The staff had been expecting the worst at any time, as he'd had a temporal operation that morning, and had not yet recovered consciousness. Studying his bed-ticket in the cabin first, I then silently entered between the screens that surrounded his bed. Only twenty-two and not even on his own soil weighted my heart. The little I could see of all that was left visible, from a large pure white turban of bandages and cotton-wool, gave me the impression there was a decent family or someone, hoping and waiting for his return. Man had pitched in all his skill on this delicate op. and now no-one but God, could determine his destiny. Silently praying with all the reverance at my command, I pleaded from my heart that he be allowed to at least get home. As the silence of night gradually wore on, he still just lay there unresponsive to my taking his T.P.R. (Temperature, Pulse and Respiration) every quarter of an hour. His expected time came and went without a movement. When my relief came for me to go to supper, I did not want to go nor even felt hungry. I wanted to see this boy come round. With his temperature down to 95, and his respirations which were very hard to take dropped to 10, his pulse-rate at only 44, and midnight had come and gone, I still did not want to leave, nor could they convince me I must have a break. The long vigil lost its tension, when at two a.m. he slowly opened his eyes and asked, "What's the time nurse?" I seemed conscious of my whole mind and body relaxing as he quietly spoke, and felt my prayers had been answered. He would go home to his people.

The following morning as the day staff came on duty, one nurse asked what time I had to lay him out, and was almost shocked with surprise to see him sitting up having a cup of tea

Sleep almost overtook me before I had reached my cabin. Feeling like a new pin as I went on duty that night, I found I had very little to do. One of the other nurses and I decided to curl up on two armchairs, so that we could peep through the crack we had left in the screens, and guard each other in between Sister's rounds. So that we get some sleep and be able to go ashore next day. The arrangement was that Marion slept for the first two hours. This went off very well, but having had such a good rest that day I could not sleep, but Marion had not and really proved it. On Sister's early morning round Marion did not respond to my elephant whisper, so I pushed her with my foot and she thought old nick had her, when without meaning to, I had pushed so hard she sailed into a patient's bed, chair and all.

The rest of the month was very happy, and between us we managed quite a lot of sleep. I spent most of my days ashore, and headed straight for the New Zealand club. I knew even if it were empty Nana and Van would be there. For a change I would go along to the New Zealand association to help Mrs. Ferguson out with a bit of typing. She did a sterling job in organising entertainment and outings for the Kiwis.

On the eleventh of August, Gracie Fields was to appear in person in the Sydney Showgrounds. Night-duty or no night-duty, I was not going to miss this exceptionally grand trouper with a heart of gold, who, though not known to us personally, together with George Formby, were part of us in their own spheres.

Towards the end of my nights, word came through that Japan had surrendered. Within a few hours it was proved to be false. The next day word went round again that it was true, but once again it was proved to be false. When I had finished my nights I went to Nana's for my three day stand off. The following morning with the sun streaming into my room Nana woke me to tell me that peace had been declared, and had a small drink of wine in her hand to drink to peace. Hardly opening my eyes, I sleepily announced, "I've heard that story before, I'm still tired," and turned over to finish my dream.

"It's really true Mona, here's a glass of wine to celebrate." Still disbelieving I sat up, and as I did so I could hear once again all the hooters, sirens, car-horns, whistles and anything at all that could make a noise, fill the air with their ceaseless blowing. "Now do you believe me Mona?" smiled Nana.

"Yes Nana I do," and to her I drank to peace, but in my heart I drank for the safety of someone else, as there were still mines to dodge on the high seas.

Breakfast was a very hurried affair, and I had to walk to town along with hundreds of others heading in the same direction. Everyone was dancing in the streets as I made my way to the New Zealand club. Van was already there serving tea, so I gave her a hand as she could hardly keep pace with it. Talking laughing and high spirits continued all day. In the evening as the boys had left the club to go on board of one of the ships tied up in the harbour to celebrate, I left the club to go back to Nana's. Shortly after leaving the club, in the distance I could hear some Kiwis really giving a haka a fair dinkum airing. As soon as they were close enough I joined them as I knew them all. With the legs of their pants rolled up, wearing piu-pius they had made from straw, we continued on with our happy singing till 1a.m. Nana didn't mind a bit when I got in, and promised not to wake me next morning.

That afternoon I went to the association to help Mrs. Ferguson, as I felt like doing some typing. She had arranged for a party of sixty-four Kiwis to go on a sight-seeing tour to the Blue Mountains the following day. They wanted me to go too, but I couldn't as I was due back at the hospital, so I suggested that Mrs. Ferguson seek permission for me to be able to go with them, as I felt that I had been in hot water long enough. She did, and it was granted.

The following day we filled two buses, and left for a most interesting time. Half way there, we stopped to stretch our legs. After a spell, as we were boarding the buses again, we discovered eight of the boys were missing. Everyone turned to search for them. Eventually they were located lying flat on their stomachs, watching a family of snakes in a snake-pit. Arriving at Katoomba we were to be welcomed with a civic reception. Since we had arrived earlier than expected, a few of the boys decided on a quick drink, as it was so hot. It was a very embarrassing moment, when we all had to slip in just after the reception had commenced, being the only girl in uniform made it even worse.

The kind hospitality shown to us all was never to be forgotten. The out-cropping of rock, towering high above

Jamieson Valley, known as the Three Sisters, crowned the beauty of the Blue Mountains. The sensational almost perpendicular drop nearly to the bottom of Jamieson Valley, in an open scenic railway car, proved to be the highlight of a wonderful day. Australia did have outstanding preserved beauty, in her vast bush lands.

On our arrival back we went first to the British Club in Hyde Park for tea, and then on to our club for a New Zealand dance. Sitting in the lounge-room of the club, I returned my now lively Kiwi's companionship on the train by wanting to fall asleep. I felt so drowsy, that I had to leave. The spectacular drop in the car that afternoon had not affected me for some time after the men.

I was delighted to find my next duty was on the Wren's ward. We had a lovely Sister, and the whole atmosphere was light and happy. Friday night dances at the New Zealand club, were now a must for me. I very soon gained the co-operation of the Wren's in helping me to slip out. I did not have to get up so early either. Rising at 7.55 a.m. I would throw my bedclothes up in a semblance of having made my bed, fling my uniform on, run a comb through my hair, and race across to be on the ward by 8 a.m. Once there, I could slip into their bathroom to wash and groom up. The delicious toasted sandwiches, made a worthwhile waiting for breakfast at morning tea-time. On Friday evenings, I would take my outdoor uniform with me, and as soon as Sister went off duty, change in their bathroom, with one up-patient watching to see the coast by the ramp was clear. One by the bathroom door would let me know, and one would close the door at the far end of the ward, after I had slipped out into the darkness, to wend my way round the maze of wards to the main gate. By some sheer gift of good fortune, I was always able to get a stand-in, when I was supposed to be on duty, and not one Wren let out our secret.

Work became slack, when we had to clear the wards as much as possible, to wait for the first arrival of P.O.W.s.

One afternoon Sister asked me to serve up the lunch. Liquid diets, light diets, salt-free diets, and so on had to be carefully considered. I could not understand why there was so little sauce for the steamed pudding. Having sucessfully completed my job of serving lunch, making the sauce spin out, I was mildly surprised to see the patients all coming back. I had put the salad dressing on them all. No one complained in that happy ward.

Just as I was about to leave the ward, Brad, an S.B.A. stuck his head round the galley door and asked "Have you seen the light Kiwi?"

"What light?" I enquired. "Oh not again!" I gasped. Grabbing screens, I screened off all strict-bed patients, and the rest disappeared, out of sight. They had come to dread the presence of a representative of some religious organisation, who was forcing her doctrine on them. Our patients represented a very wide range of religions, each respecting each other. As we did not wish to offend our visitor, we dodged her. Once she had left we settled down again. Tidying the ward before I went off duty, I rearranged all the flowers. Walking in with a vase, Sister stopped me and asked me to alter them as red and white flowers together in a vase, was a long standing superstition of a death in the ward. Respecting her wishes, I did as I was asked.

As very heavy footsteps approached our ward, I went to see who it was. One of the doctors had wanted to get his horse Nelson across the ground in a hurry and was leading him in a short cut through all the ramps.

Once off duty I went straight to the club and was amazed not to find Nana and Van there, but a crowd of Kiwis. Then I remembered it was Thursday the day the men had the club to themselves. As I apologised and was about to leave, Colonel

133

Patterson invited me to share a drink, declaring I was the only woman member of their club. Meeting Vera later on my way back to the hospital, we found we had much in common as we had both been to Haslar. She told me she had met another New Zealand V.A.D. while she was there. I wished that I had met her. Later we discovered we were at Haslar together and were both surprised to find it was me, only now I was almost three stone lighter.

Soon the hospital-ship 'Oranje' arrived in Sydney. Our wards were almost empty, and we had been having a pretty easy time. While having afternoon tea, the first P.O.W.s began to arrive. As I looked up the ramp to where they were coming down towards our ward, I had never in my life witnessed such a heart-rending horrible sight. How any human being could possibly survive in such a state of deplorable malnutrition, and sheer neglect, is beyond human comprehension. A surge of hatred rose and subsided as each emaciated individual either walked, or was helped, or was borne on a stretcher towards us. No human being could possibly allow such suffering even to the lowliest of creatures. I could not believe my eyes. My God it isn't possible that they are really still alive, stuck in my throat.

With a weeping heart, and tears burning the backs of my eyes, I silently and unnoticed slipped behind the galley door. The relief to sob and hide my tears made me feel very ashamed to be called a nurse. Surely I had more courage than this. Our heroic Maori Battalion didn't run away, and weep behind a galley door, when they were outnumbered thirty-three to one on Crete. No. They did a war haka and faced their enemy, and made them literally run for their lives. Our Maori is a natural born, fearless warrior, with great heroic courage, making him a formidable enemy. Our New Zealanders too, earned their great popularity and respect, so must I. Determinedly summoning my self-control, I was sandwiched in by my colleague, who broke down too. Smiling at each other through our tears, we egged each other on to start work, but neither of us moved. Before we had time to re-appear, Sister called us as she peeped round the door. With misty sad eyes "I'm coming too," she whispered. "In all my years of nursing, and I have had some shocking cases, I have never seen anything like this in all my life," she quietly told us. Comforted by her sincere natural understanding, we suppressed our emotional shock and began with our usual calm efficiency, which had developed over the years, to receive our pathetically wasted patients.

Tucking in one patient who just stared glassily at every move I made, I learned she had an abdominal cancer, and had suffered excrutiating pain for six months, with no drugs or treatment what-so-ever. Not even any proper food to give her a few moments respite. Her condition was so serious, there was no hope of optimistic speculation, and was transferred after a rest later that same afternoon to a civilian hospital, where she died a fortnight later. Her one wish was to hang on, until she got to her own soil, and was granted that wish.

Many bore the tell-tale marks of inhuman acts of sadism. Many broke down just to see the long forgotten comfort of white sheets, to rest their exhausted bodies between. It was impossible to comprehend how they had survived. One felt so desolate and inadequate, as for so long they had been completely deprived of relief or palliation. Into our sympathetic ears poured many tragic stories. The Red Cross emblazoned on the bib of our spotless white aprons, signifying our status, put us on a pedestal to them. Many of their eyes filled with tears. While still in captive hands most had openly wept, just to see the Union Jack hoisted again. "Oh nurse you are so kind and gentle," fell on most our ears, touching our hearts very deeply, as we were only doing the job we had joined up to do.

Immediately after all the patients had been made as comfortable as possible, we made them afternoon tea. There was an Australian Nursing Sister on her own in one of the small cabins, reserved for S.C.L.s (Serious Case List). As usual I set up a tray for her, and found a flower to add to it. Speaking to her as I walked in, she began weeping. Enquiring what was wrong, with great effort to control her feelings, she explained, "It's so nice nurse, to have a cup of tea from a cup and saucer. It's four years, since I've seen a cup we only had dirty rusty old tins, sometimes filled with holes to drink from." I sat on her bed, against all rules and talked to her for some time. She was such a darling. As we talked I reflected in amongst all the unspeakable horror I had just witnessed, had the Japanese landed in my own beloved New Zealand this wasted pathetic lovely person could so easily have been my own mother. No amount of abnormal privations had even scratched the surface, of the gentle, calm understanding, and patient resignation these human wrecks, whose courage, and determination had left nothing to be desired. When she was eventually discharged, she invited me to have dinner with her and her sister at the Arcadia Hotel in Sydney. We kept in touch until she died two years later.

At an invitation from the opposite ward, I went to see a baby that had been born on the hospital-ship, and was amazed to see how fit it's mother was.

Leaving the ward next day, to collect the lunch from the main galleys I noticed too, that there were a lot of New Zealanders amongst them. In a passive way they wandered about, with a glassy look in their eyes, and some seemed so vacant. Some were yellow from atebrin, and some were fat and flabby from beri-beri. I wanted to speak to them all, and tell them that 'The Land of the Long White Cloud' was still the most wonderful country in the world. Pity, anger, hatred and fear surged through my whole body. Pity for the unnecessary deplorable suffering, these one time normal people had been forced to suffer, many of whom were our nation's one time finest, fittest and best men. Many of whom I knew would never ever feel the great blessing of robust health again. Anger that such sadistical brutality should have been so wantonly administered to such one time useful people. Hatred that any nation should have acquired through sheer lack of common decency and respect the free right to massacre, and torture, as their warped minds wished, and fear, that without the courage, tenacity and phenomenal tolerance and suffering that these heroic, and gallant prisoners had portrayed, we could so easily have also been in their shoes. It made one feel ashamed to allow a furtive deep emotional sympathy to show itself, when to exercise kindness, understanding, and a will to accept this as the final phase of our struggle for freedom.

I could not transfer to the New Zealand forces, but I wanted to do all I could in my own small way for them. Slowly an idea came to me.

Finishing that day's duty, I went straight to the receiving office and asked for all the names and ward numbers of all the Kiwis that had been admitted. I skipped tea and went straight to visit each one. To be amongst human humans was miracle enough, but a real live Kiwi was too good to be true. Long question and answer sessions ensued, as I had been home so recently. "Look Kiwi to hell with your real name, a Kiwi's a Kiwi and that's that!" came from one. Giving me his wife's address, he asked me to write to her, as he could not. "Tell her I'm fit and well, and will be home soon."

Humbled by their cheerful optimism, I wondered what kind of a shock, some of their relatives would receive. Some I knew would need medical and mental treatment for an unknown time. Some were still clinging to the remaining

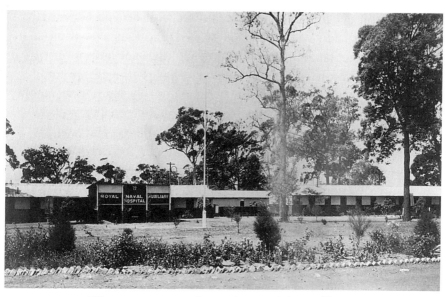

The entrance to the main receiving office.

fragments of sanity. Some would just sit for hours, and simply stare into space, often unresponsive to verbal contact. Many were hungry for New Zealand papers and magazines. For this I wrote to Mrs. North, who promptly replied she would arrange to have them sent over.

I knew the comforting joy of talking to Kiwis when away from home, and was thrilled I had plucked up enough courage to visit them all.

Heading straight for the club next afternoon to fulfil an engagement of giving a talk to its members, I told them about the boys. From then on many of the women, baked simple cakes, as the patient's shrunken stomachs could not accommodate anything rich. They too collected magazines, and visited their own countrymen. While there I was introduced to Audrey and Betty, and three other members of a dancing group, who, though trained in Sydney, had almost mastered the art of Maori action songs and dances to perfection. They entertained, when and wherever they were asked, whether it was a floor show, a hospital appearance, or even in the prisons.

They were to appear at the British Forces Club the following night.

Naturally I went with a crowd, it was a great joy to hear, and see them in traditional constume, commencing their programme with *'Karangatia-Ra'* the Maori traditional welcome song, and perfectly performing *'Hoea-Ra-Te-Waka'*, a very lovely canoe poi. Jane too, enhanced the evening with her beautiful rendering of *'This is the Story of a Starry Night'*.

The following day, I found I had been transferred to the Officer's ward. "You'll have to behave yourself on that ward" said one of my patients. As I wistfully smiled at her she thoughtfully remarked, "I wish you were staying here."

"So do I," I replied "I can't wash and change and fly off duty there, but still it's only next door so I'll pop in and see you now and again," I smiled hopefully.

139

Next day it was tragic to see the mess that some of the patients were in. Twenty-two of them were strict-bed. There were only two nurses on duty, and Sister worked ceaselessly. I worked as I had never worked before. One job dovetailing into the next with no let-up. On the second day I was fully in my stride. When lunch was over in the ward, and I had ploughed through countless dishes, I made an immediate start on the blanket baths, as there were so many to do. While I was speedily walking down the centre of the ward with a bowl of water and a tooth-mug in my hands, an up patient ready to go ashore stopped me with a glass in his hand, and affectedly asked me to get him a drink of water. Taken aback I looked straight at him. Without thinking, "Sir I am a nurse not a waitress," slipped from my lips.

The junior officer smartly cut in, "I'll report you for insubordination." A hush fell on the whole ward.

Still clutching my bowl of water and the tooth-mug, "Yours is the inconsiderate, disrespectful type, who uses his gold-braid to encourage resentment instead of respect," I wanted to retort aloud, and the strong desire to throw my bowl of water over him, nearly got the better of me. Instead, for the second time I reminded him that I was a nurse not a waitress, and left him standing in the middle of the ward, while I carried on to do what I had set out to.

True enough there was a notice on the board, requesting me to report to Matron next morning. While standing waiting my turn, I was reminded of the last time I was here was when I returned from furlough. Without giving a thought as to what might happen and responding to her come in, quite unconcerned I replied to her natural 'Good-morning'.

Her placid, calm, serenity was befitting for one whose responsibilities were great. Where tact and understanding were the keynote for the happy smooth running efficiency of the nursing staff in this vast hospital.

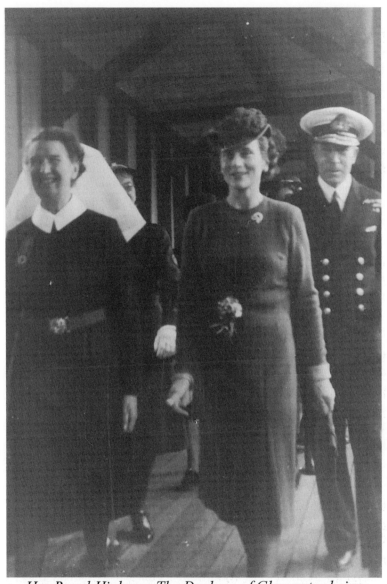

Her Royal Highness The Duchess of Gloucester being escorted round our hospital by our Matron and Surgeon Rear Admiral

She had received a complaint from one of the patients on the officer's ward and wanted an explanation. With deliberate accuracy, I openly explained in my own words what had happened. Showing no change in her countenance, "You realise nurse, you are junior to an officer," she reminded me, putting me at ease, and I felt the whole thing was too ridiculous to be made an issue of.

"Yes Matron," I replied, "but I still think my strict-bed patients are more important."

"I'm afraid you won't be able to remain on that ward," she advised me. Almost before she had finished speaking I requested to go back on the wren's ward.

"Alright nurse, report straight back there, and tell Sister I sent you," she answered, and seemed quite pleased at my request. "Most of my nurses prefer the men's wards, and so few want the wren's ward," she smiled as I left her office.

My heart skipped for joy, as I light-heartedly walked along the ramps back to 210. Once again I could slip out every Friday night, to be asked by the guards at the gate, "Have you a late pass Kiwi?"

"No, but I won't be late if I can help it," I would happily smile back continuing on my way to catch the train to Wynyard Station, making my way to the club, where I could forget the hospital atmosphere and the routine, to enjoy the happy jovial company I always found there.

When I appeared back on the wren's ward, I was promptly greeted with, "Not you again so soon, didn't you like it next door?" Really happy to be back, I told them what had happened, which attracted many wry smiles and comments of, "We won't see you on Friday nights again."

"Not if I can help it," I replied. "That's why I'm so glad to be back."

"You win Kiwi, but one day you'll get caught, and then you really will be in trouble," warned one.

"I'll deserve it if I do, but I'll still take the chance and wait until that day comes." My mischief didn't last long, as I was transferred to ward 119.

In amongst the patients was an Indian who could not speak any English. The whole atmosphere was such a vast change from the wren's ward. The patients erred on the cheeky rather uncouth side. While sprucing the ward for rounds one morning, I was advised that it had fallen to me to follow the round's party with each patient's bed-ticket. When our much respected and well loved Surgeon Rear Admiral asked the Indian how he was, he smiled back and answered with the only English words he had been taught, which were the crudest and most undesirable I ever had the misfortune to hear. The obvious embarrassment and disgust of the round's party raised self-satisfied smiles from the low sense of humour of the apparent culprits. For the first time since I had joined up I questioned my sincere attempts to do my best; to assist in helping these men back on their feet. I felt as though every ounce of enthusiasm and genuine effort was flung back in my face. I was thankful when my duty on that ward had finished, as it made me feel I could no longer give of my best for such contemptible ignorance; but remembered the friendly cards and letters I seemed always privilaged to receive from so many patients, both men and women whom I had once nursed. I thought also of the next-of-kin; friends and relations back home, who would be praying and waiting for the boys overseas to return home. Of the great brilliant and intelligent men and women of all nationalities, who had already made real sacrifices in the cause for freedom. Regaining my original desire to fulfill my chosen war-time occupation, I continued on as before.

Luck was in my path once again as I was soon back on the wren's ward. How I loved that ward. It always seemed to have lovely understanding Sisters. I enjoyed talking to Lillian

143

during slack moments, as she was one of the very few V.A.D.s who landed in sick-bay for an op. Also lovely Susan who, while sight-seeing around Sydney, slipped on some rocks and fractured both her ankles. We teased her about a two-piece nightdress she made, and later declared it was never any good anyway.

One morning while I was making toasted sandwiches as fast as possible, a Kiwi came to the ward to see me. "We're on our way back home Kiwi, and we've come to say Goodbye." The toast burnt as I talked to the sixteen men that had arrived. Someone else took over my job while we talked. As they were not leaving till early evening, I rang Audrey to see if we could give them a proper New Zealand send off. When they left Sister gave me back my job and smiled, "I thought the whole New Zealand Navy was coming up." What an understanding and sporting person she was.

That evening Audrey and the girls turned up, and it almost made me want to weep, when along with all the others, we sang *'Now is the Hour'* as the ship slowly slipped from her moorings, and silently moved away, taking with her the first of my wonderful companions, who were singing with us from the ship, until distance made their voices fade right away. There is no tune as touching, sincere, or beautiful, as *'Now is the Hour'* sung in either Maori or English, while a majestic ship glides gracefully out to sea.

I was invited out by one of the remaining Kiwis, as we turned to leave the wharf. Feeling rather sad I told him, "I would rather go with a crowd."

"There is someone else?" he ventured.

"Yes," I told him.

"When will you see him again?" he enquired.

"I don't know. The last I heard from him, he had been transferred on to the *Implacable* and was trying to get here." I managed to confide in him. I had been becoming increasingly worried, as for reasons unknown to me, I had received no replies to my mail for some time.

After a long thoughtful pause he replied, "O.K. Kiwi, I'll see you at the dance as usual." When he left I felt very saddened, but as there was still so much to do, I had no time to figure out why.

I soon found myself taking my turn on nights again. Gayly arriving on my allotted ward I found a nurse already there. So tried another two wards before finding one without a nurse. I read bed-tickets and the day-report, until the night Sister confirmed my ward for me. Most of the patients were P.O.W's and in very good spirits. Having reached the convalescent stage, they were not in the deplorable state that so many of the others still were. Quite a number had been repatriated home, and most of the others had gone ashore to see them off and to celebrate. It was getting very close to round's time before they returned, and all were very merry. They were all singing and fooling around like a pack of kids. What was I going to do with them, I didn't want them to get caught, and I certainly didn't want to report them for being late. Talking was hopeless, warning them of how late it was, was just as hopeless, so I let out an almighty yell, *"ROUNDS!!"* As it resounded right round the ward they all jumped to it, but hadn't enough time to change, so hurriedly scrambled into bed, boots and all. As the dignified round's party passed down the ward speaking casually to each patient, my heart raced madly, in case any of the uniforms were not properly hidden by the bed-clothes, I had great difficulty in not bursting into laughter, as every patient that had been spoken too giggled to himself, causing his blankets to vibrate with his endeavours to control his own merry mirth. What a relief it was to get away with it, and what a mad scramble to change before anyone else appeared on the ward.

The following week I was guest of honour at a gathering in Martin Place. Noho Toki was to sing a solo, and to do a haka. With his exceptionally fine voice he sang *'Because'*. Then in his traditional costume, and carrying a green-stone miri, he went into a very lively spirited haka. Half way through his item, a mongrel dog began to yap at his heels. When Noho really got going, he finished up by jumping high in the air off the impromptu stage, and landed close to the dog. With a yelp it took off at top speed! I believe that this fine Maori chief could trace his ancestry back over 600 years. Later in the day I had to address a meeting of Australian Red Cross members, before going on to my usual Friday night dance.

When I arrived there was only one Kiwi there. "Now I can dance with you all night Kiwi," he teased.

"No jolly fear, you forget there's a floor to dance on," I teased back. Jokingly I suggested that we go and find some men. Then it dawned on me there was a dance on in the British Club in Hyde Park.

"Where Kiwi?" he asked.

"If you'll come with me I'll show you," I smiled filled with mischievousness. Descending the stairs, leaving puzzled smiles on the faces of the few girls in the club, we left. "You'll get me shot Kiwi," he protested as I led him towards the British club.

"Let's join in the dance, and collar any Kiwi we see," I suggested.

It was fun. As we danced and noticed a New Zealand flash, my partner jokingly asked what he thought he was doing. Bewildered they asked what he meant. "There's a Kiwi dance on and no men; come on!" In this way, we found only five. That wasn't enough. One of them with a sense of devilry suggested crocodiling back to Bridge Street. singing *'Maori Battalion'* followed by a very great favourite *'Pokarekare'*,

146

made so famous by our own lovely singer Ana Hato, and of course *'Waita Poi'* and many others, our crocodile began to grow. Passing along a main street, we held our breaths as Kiwis on trams who heard us, simply leapt off, dodging the heavy traffic to find out what it was all about. By the time we reached Bridge Street. we had collected 28 men, and heartily sang as we mounted the stairs at the club, *'E Pari Ra,'* which is the Maori farewell song, dedicated to the boys of the First World War. Others had arrived while we were away, and the high spirited gay hilarity carried on non-stop for the rest of the night, with the *'Notre Dam March'* being a very great favourite, and requested time after time.

Time was slipping by and I was soon back on the wren's ward again. Half way through one morning, three Kiwis came racing down on to the ward and surprised me. "Kiwi the *Implacable's* berthed," they breathed aloud together.

"What?" I almost yelled. Excited I thanked them. I could not concentrate nor wait for him to get shore leave. At long last I could at least have a chance to sort out our problems and find out why there had been such a long silence. Three hours later, the same three Kiwis returned like gentlemen for a change, and apologised for having made a mistake, as it was the *Indefatigable* that had berthed. My heart sank so low, but there was still hope, as the *Implacable* was expected in Sydney. Three weeks later when she did arrive, he was not on board. I did not understand there was still no mail, nor any replies to my letters. What had happened? Only God knew, even if I couldn't understand. I could only conclude perhaps it just wasn't meant to be.

ONE OF MANY

After duty that day, I sat in Jane's cabin, quietly chatting as she was packing for her redraft to Hong Kong. I had not put my name down for this draft. The fear of being caught in England again was too forbidding, as I knew that shipping would be very limited for a long time to come after the war. Around 9 p.m. a message was brought to me, that there was someone waiting to see me. With a dull empty feeling, with no cap, or belt on, my blue uniform hung loosely from my shoulders, as I strolled along the ramp to see who it was.

I was surprised to see one of the Kiwis at this hour of the night, who suggested that I go up to a small cafe known as Smokey Jo's for a cup of coffee. Not feeling at all up to the mark, I excused myself, but he insisted that I come, as he had something to tell me. "I don't know how to tell you Kiwi," and seemed rather concerned.

"What's happened?" I asked him.

"I'm afraid Kiwi, that you will never hear from your friend again." Literally stunned and dazed, I thanked him. My heart grew so heavy that it made me feel speechless. All my gaiety and happy hope, that some day we would meet again, fled completely, as though it were a myth anyway. A film began to mist my eyes as I slowly made my way to my own cabin. It just seemed that instead of still hoping that one day all my troubles would be little ones, they were cascading down in torrents as though bent on destroying my very soul, and every moment of happiness I had ever known. The sincere strains of *'We'll Meet Again'* that always boosted my morale, when time seemed to drag, became cruel torment. Or was it just the exposure of a secret hidden fear so many of us carried in our hearts, of loved ones away on active service, which we glossed over to enable us to work efficiently and cheerfully. Perhaps one day I may know the truth of what happened, but who am I to question my destiny.

Our hearts are ever truthful, no matter what turmoil we have to face, and must not procrastinate on the rough patches in life, but only face and accept them as God's will.

I had witnessed heartbreak and grief so often in my patients and colleagues, but had never realised before the severe overwhelming and desolate impact it placed on one's heart and soul. I consoled myself, that I was only one of many. One must expect heartbreak in war, and should never have a heart of feeling, but treat all contacts, as we are, just one number in a very large number of numbers with a job to do, irrespective of creed, class, colour, nationality or rank. The war had become too personal for me now, and one should give orders where demanded, and accept them without question or individual initiative or ambition.

As I entered my cabin my eyes fell on the photo that was always waiting for me when I came off duty, smiling so sincerely from the frame I had managed to get in Auckland on my furlough, made more appropriate by the naval crest. Soon it began to swim, and as my head and hands sank deeper and deeper into the side of my bed, I felt I was slowly being mystically carried away and wished that I would never return.

Too exhausted and broken, I remained fully clothed on the top of my bedclothes, ignoring my room-mate's insistence I should wash and change. So typical of British understanding when occasion demands, she woke me from an exhausted sleep next morning, and showed no emotion at my unexpected flood of tears that came from nowhere, and from a depth I didn't know I had. "It's got to be a mistake!" I sobbed.

Once on the wards assisting to alleviate the sufferings caused by inhuman treachery, I felt thoroughly ashamed for allowing my own personal misfortune to take command of my will and struggled to put my patients first.

Work seemed to go on just as usual, but for no reason, even while I was working, I kept wanting to break down but could not. My patients needed a cheerful nurse. I found that I could not keep pace with the cheerful chiding and backchat, that made the atmosphere so happy for both the nurses and the patients alike. To escape from letting myself down, I periodically took a couple of unimportant papers from Sister's desk, and wandered round the hospital, as I didn't dare go to my cabin. As I walked I wondered was I fortunate in not having come to a decision. I thought of Norma who had lost her infant, of the nurse at the Gables who had lost her husband, and of so many many others, who had the courage I did not to marry during the war.

Automaton seemed to set in, so I was still able to work. Food became tasteless and would not go down. All I could take was snacks off the ward. Somehow I just couldn't be cheered, even by the Kiwis who had been such wonderful cobbers for so long. Even the Jewel of the South Seas had lost it's lustre for me.

The following Sunday when I went to church, as I slowly and thoughtfully mounted the steps, the shimmering heat mercilously beat down, creating a blinding glare, reflected from the white of the wide concrete steps. Once in the coolness inside, my reverence was stabilised as I glanced up at the crucifix behind the altar. The choir seemed extra beautiful that day, giving me a feeling of inner comfort and peace, without detracting from serene thought. As I knelt to pray, the solitary plane that droned overhead ironically in peace time, did not detract from the one thought I had in mind.

After church I felt I could not go to any of my friend's places, as I would be no company for them. I did not want sympathy, as I felt it would be an encroachment on something very exclusive. I did not wish to speak to anyone. I felt so alone wrapped in my own thoughts, as though I was out of this world so went along to the Cook's river. Stepping from the train into the sun that blazed down from a cloudless sky, to scorch the earth beneath it, I was soon in a world where the unending, though shrill, grating chirruping of countless thousands of giant cicadas, brought comfort. The dirty huge yellow jellyfish, that floated aimlessly in the Cook's river, and the giant trees with an uneven rim of golden giant cicada's shells, transmitted a feeling of restfulness.

As I sat on a bench in the shade of the trees, I consoled myself I was not the only one, and thought of that lovely card from Bill, and didn't realise till then, just how very true it was. How long I stayed there I do not know. I began to think of my patients, their plight was far worse than mine, some irreparable. Gradually they took command of my thoughts, my spirit, and only my patients mattered now. Slowly and thoughtfully I boarded the next train back to Herne Bay.

Night duty was soon round again. Following taking over from the day staff, I found I had several penicillin injections to give, otherwise no treatments. Entering the ward with the treatment tray, I was asked if I played darts. Smiling roguishly I said "No."

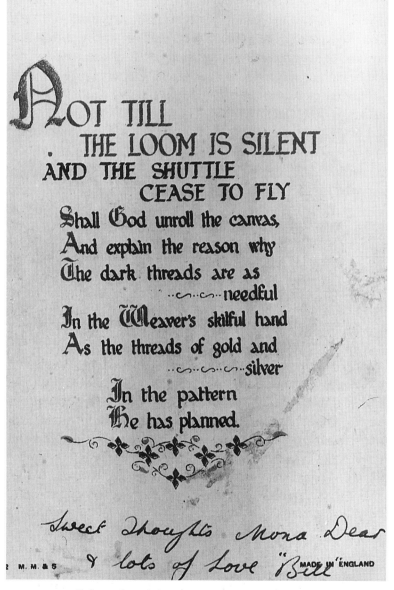

Not Till
THE LOOM IS SILENT
AND THE SHUTTLE
CEASE TO FLY
Shall God unroll the canvas,
And explain the reason why
The dark threads are as
··········· needful
In the Weaver's skilful hand
As the threads of gold and
············silver

In the pattern
He has planned.

*Sweet Thoughts Mona Dear
& lots of Love "Bill"*

I thought of that lovely card from Bill.

"The day staff practises on us," they said. I couldn't help bubbling over with laughter. They really seemed a happy crowd. On the completion of my round of injections, "She'll do us boys, she's champion, I didn't feel a thing," accompanied me from the ward, as I blithely wondered how many other nurses had heard the same words.

When I went to put the lights out at nine, I was surprised to find that every patient that could, squatting on the end of his bed. Perplexed I shrugged my shoulders, and reached for the light cords. Then I knew why. Every light cord was twisted over the bare wooden rafters. "Whoever put those light cords up, can put the lights out," I reproved mildly.

"Oh nurse be a sport," came in the chorus. "We paid five bob a seat just to watch you do it." I wasn't going to play cheap cheesecake, flashed through my mind, I'd had a lot of fun joining in many a prank, and turning a blind eye to many that others would have reported, but this to my mind was a bit much. When the round's party was in the next ward, I asked them again to put the lights out as it was now after nine, but they just sat there. "You know you'll get it, if the lights aren't out nurse," they all chorused again.

"You'll know you'll get it too, when they know why," I happily answered them. Quite satisfied I would remain adamant, when the S.B.A. from the rounds's party arrived on the ward, all the lights went out as if by magic and every man was in bed.

They really were a happy crowd. Going back to the quarters one morning, my heart dropped, more nurses were being drafted to hospital-ships, and some were going on to the *Implacable*. I was not to be one of them. Perhaps the hand of Providence had decreed that I should never have that wish granted.

As soon as shipping space became available, as many patients as possible were repatriated. There was still so much to do, that I'd had no time to allow the mental strain of not knowing what had happened catch up with me.

It was almost too good to be true to be back on the wren's ward, after finishing my nights. For some unknown reason I was finding it hard to keep pace with all my work. It was annoying as the great rush had lessened and so many patients had been repatriated, as well as some of the V.A.D.s. On my weekend off, I went to stay with some friends, hoping to regain my usual enthusiasm. After lunch a large group of us went down to Cooggee beach for the afternoon. Racing onto the beach along with all the others, I flung my towel down and flopped on it as we all did, but four hours later they woke me to go home for tea. That evening they had an informal party, and the last I remembered was someone playing the piano for a hearty sing-song. Late next morning I woke up in my hostess's bed, having collapsed at the party from sheer exhaustion.

Reporting for duty after my weekend away, I could not somehow summon any energy, and was becoming increasingly dogged by exhaustion, and forced to spend more and more time aboard. I had already made inquiries, and found that the Berlitz School of Languages taught the course I wanted to study, so that I could get started as soon as I was discharged. I had been informed that as soon as I had reached a certain standard I could go into the rehabilitation class, and after completing my course, would go on to Melbourne for two years for experience, and then transfer to Singapore as I wished to do.

I tried to keep going, bearing in mind, I could not go sick now, as there were still many patients who needed the little I could do for them.

Xmas was coming up again, and I had arranged with Audrey and the girls to entertain on the wards. They always gave their time freely and willingly, and their items were well worth seeing and hearing. I had discovered with shock, that Lyn had collapsed on night duty, and was in isolation on the wren's ward, with T.B. affecting both lungs. Audrey and the girls gave of their best, on Xmas Eve, and their rendering of *Pakete Whero*, a very lively poi, and *Toia Mai Te Waka*, which was dedicated to the treaty of Waitangi, brought us great joy. They stayed on extra long for Lyn's sake, as she enjoyed it so much.

On a slack afternoon, in order to keep going, I lay on the couch in the examining room. Unfortunately Sister breezed in before I could slip out. We had not been so fortunate this time, as she was one of the very few who was very provocative, and hurled something at me from her sharp tongue. Unable to exercise the calm control a nurse must have, and refusing to submit, or admit to my malady, I too burst forth at her. This landed me in sick-bay, instead of Matron's office. Being query T.B. myself now and only weighing 6st.12ozs. I was permitted to remain in my quarters. A fine kettle of fish when there was still New Zealanders to visit. Coming through the tests as negative, they tested for anaemia. This too proved not the complaint, but with something wrong somewhere, I was assigned to quarters duty where I could rest, but had to report periodically for check-ups.

On quarters duty and plenty of time to rest, I did not realise till then just how very tired I was. Apart from visiting New Zealanders still in hospital I did not even feel like going ashore. I began not to care if I went on duty again or not. Even my wonderful Friday nights at the club, seemed not to encourage me.

Mail from the friends I had made were a blessing in disguise. One letter; 'Dear Kiwi, I'm in trouble, please come to ward 119," and signed, made me pull myself together. Answering his request, I found he was being repatriated home, and that his uniform had ripped. I repaired it for him before he left for New Zealand. Letters of a similar nature I always attended to first. They were my life. I will be eternally grateful to my

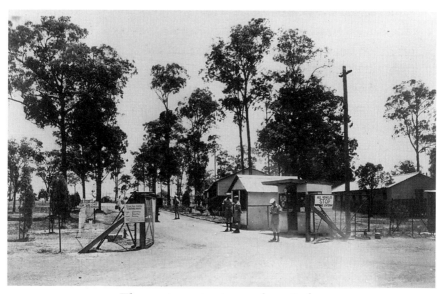

The main gates to our hospital.

parents, who opened their home, and gave some of my South Island boys a bed for the night, before going on the rest of their long journey, after arriving in Auckland.

After about a month, I began to pick up, and started unofficially going ashore. It wasn't quite so easy to by-pass the powers that be, when I should have been aboard, as our members had depleted with so many being re-drafted, and repatriated. The same guards were still on the gate, and now they asked, "Are you supposed to be ashore?"

Occcassionally it was yes. One afternoon as I gayly went to pass through the gate, the answer was "No".

They remarked "Watch it Wiggy's behind you, get in the guard hut." Fortunately our Commandant was still too far behind to have seen me, and once in the hut, I was pushed under the table, given a cigarette, and ordered not to breathe. In her usual courteous way, she spoke to the guards, while they held their breaths in case she entered the hut, as she sometimes did to use the phone. What a relief when she went straight through. Apart from not having shore leave, I was wearing silk stockings instead of my uniform ones. Missing one train, because I knew she would be on it, I really brightened up to see Nana and Van at the club again. Returning quite early two Kiwis saw me on to the train. As I was standing in the doorway, saying hooray to them, our Assistant Commandant only just caught it - and me too, wearing my silk stockings and no hat.

Next morning she confronted me with it.

"Are you sure?" I questioned as though I wouldn't do such a thing. With a kindly, knowing, understanding smile she dropped it. I had always liked Miss Pelly. More for sheer mutual companionship, she asked me to make sure our dormitory was clean and tidy for rounds. Before I had finished, the round's party was well on its way. Going like a scalded

157

cat, I swept my heap of dust under the mat in the front of the fireplace. Without saying a word, as though I wasn't there, the round's party inspected the dorm, passing their hands over the ledges and parts that we all like to miss, and standing on the mat, Matron complemented me on my work.

After three months of drifting, I was recommended for discharge on medical grounds, as I was still suffering from very severe bouts of migraine, although I did not feel anywhere as near as exhausted as I had been. Stunned into reality, I exclaimed, "I can't, I have to find employment as soon as I am discharged, so that I can study for my future." I was then tried on an easy ward. It was so hot, that your damp clothes simply stuck to you. The ward was so easy that it was very hard to keep occupied. Half asleep one afternoon from sheer heat, as we were making beds in slow motion, the radio quietly added to our lethargy. Dreaming away to a very relaxing tune, I was startled when the soothing tune burst into the famous crash of Spike Jones' *'Cocktails for two'*. My sudden jerking to life, brought spontaneous laughter from the handful of patients we had. In order to overcome our boredom, my colleague and I had a competition to see how fast we could make a bed. With our patients as time-keepers, we flew into action, and with exact precision in stripping the beds, and folding the blankets properly, and remaking the beds, we were clocked at one a minute.

Within a couple of days, I was back on nights on ward 210. There were no treatments, so I had nothing to do. We also had a very lovely Sister again. I had also been going ashore more. One of my dorm mates asked me, if she could borrow my alarm clock, as she was on nights and wanted to get up early one afternoon. I lent it to her, but on returning it, she apologised, as her mirror had fallen directly on top if it, and had indented it, otherwise it was not damaged. Not to worry,

158

I took it with me on nights, as I intended sleeping in between rounds so that I could go ashore. The first night I did this, I found the alarm would not stop ringing once it went off. Not wishing to be caught, I wrapped it in a blanket to lessen the noise. This didn't work, and as I was wrapping a second blanket round it, Sister appeared wondering what was going on. Feeling rather stupid, but bubbling over inside, at the spectacle it must have made, I admitted my intentions. Smiling brightly she said she had just awakened another nurse by giving her a fright when she tickled her nose with a feather. The following night I decided to lie on the floor wrapped in a blanket. This way I could hear her coming. After the ten o'clock round and still no treatments to do I settled down. This time I was disturbed by a very sore foot. Investigating why, I found that my foot had slowly but surely, gone further and further into the radiator, and I had already burnt the toe of my slipper.

I gave these capers up as a bad job, and just dozed off on my arms on the desk, as all my patients slept all night. A septicaemia case was admitted and required constant watching. Spending most of the night with her, she seemed more comfortable in the early hours of the morning. Sister had been in frequently as we had cause for concern. Feeling the strain a bit, I rested my head on my arms after I had written up my night report. Silently as the first light of dawn appeared and filtered through the darkness of night, as though magically taking command of the heavens for yet another stiffling hot day, I became aware of a faint sound. Making sure my S.C.L. was still alright, I left to trace the sound. Just as I stepped on the ramp, I was attracted by it again, and there, caught high up in the rafters, was a dear little tabby kitten that was completely lost. I took him back to the quarters with me, as I now had a two berth cabin, and hoped that my room mate would not mind. He was a lovely companion, and gave us hours of fun, getting into mischief.

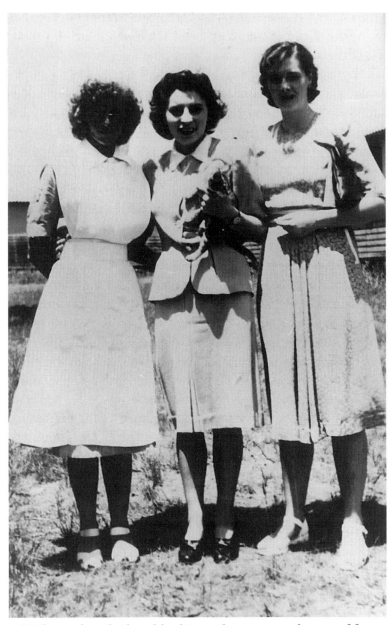

With my dear little tabby kitten that gave us hours of fun.

Some of the nurses had made pets of opposums, and hand fed them with the immense variety of fruit we had in great abundance.

My next ward was 113, which faced the road and was half empty, as so many patients had been repatriated. They were full of high spirits, and were more or less marking time, before repatriation. Being on an early shift I was off at two and was heading straight for the club. One of the Kiwis nicknamed 'Whiskers' because of his beard, was determined to accompany me there. Preferring to go alone, I told him I was not off till two, and would meet him there at three. As I was waiting for rounds, and then to go off duty, he tramped up the ramps. "You can't come on the ward I told him, as we are expecting rounds." Before he had time to leave, the round's party was already on its way. He couldn't hide in the heads (ablution blocks),as they were inspected too. Whiskers was not to be caught, so stood alongside one of the empty beds. As the round's party was passing down the wards, his flashes were noticed.

"Hello, a New Zealander?" was remarked to him.

"Yes Sir," answered Whiskers.

"Are they treating you alright?" he was asked.

"Yes Sir, very well indeed," answered Whiskers.

"When are you leaving?"

"Very shortly," he replied as the rounds party moved off. As Sister passed me, she remarked,

"I didn't know you had a New Zealander on the ward nurse, may I see his bed-ticket please?"

"He's for discharge Sister, and his bed-ticket has already been handed in," I lied with my fingers crossed.

"Alright nurse," she said as she was leaving. Phew! that was the closest shave I'd had yet and ducked off duty as fast as I could.

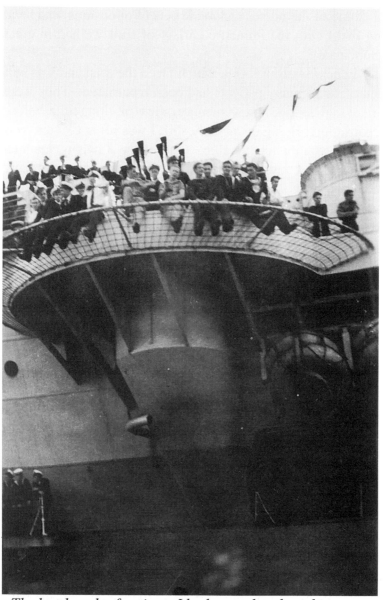

The last bunch of patients I had nursed gathered in a gun-turret, throwing ever cheerful remarks.

NOW IS THE HOUR

The day arrived when there was sufficient shipping so that the greater majority of the patients could be repatriated. I had taken out my discharge in Sydney, so that I could get started on my studies as soon as I was released, and so remained behind with a handful of staff. Fortunately I was off duty that day and went down to the docks at Woolloomooloo together with most of our nurses, to wave them off on the Aircraft carrier *'Indefatigable'*. The wharf was crowded and made gay by the countless streamers being thrown to and from the ship.

The last bunch of patients I had nursed gathered in a gun-turret throwing ever cheerful remarks.

"If you ever visit England again, Kiwi, come and visit us!" Little did they know if only circumstances were different I would have been on board with them, despite the struggle I'd had to get home. Those guards, who in their own way had done so much for me, and indeed risked being found out each time they handed my late pass in on the odd occasion, when I knew that I would be late after attending a New Zealand ball.

Slowly my heart seemed to get heavier and heavier. I carried thoughts of long hours, gaity, mischief and radiant happiness.

163

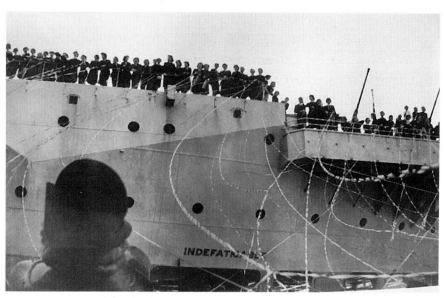

I looked up at the girls lining the deck

No one can live, work and suffer, with such fine people for so long, and share their joys, sorrows and heartaches, and not feel a genuine admiration for them all. Each one would be returning in peace, with no more partings, no more waiting.

I stood alone on the wharf, yet surrounded by so many, I knew in my heart I would never have the future and happiness that once seemed so near, but resolved to build a new life, as so many others would have to do in a peaceful but tired world, and thanked God for allowing me to come out of the war a comparatively fit person.

When the majestic ship cast off her mooring, I watched the widening space between ship and shore fill with bubbling water, created by her massive propellors, and then slowly glide towards Sydney Heads. I looked up at the girls lining the deck and the men moving to dress ship. "Good Luck, Kiwi!" once again came across the water. Slowly and silently she gradually moved further and further away, 'God Bless England!' 'Ma Te Atua Koutou Katoa E Manaaki!' in English. "God bless you all." And all who live within her shores, especially the men and women who fought, worked and died so gallantly in the Royal Navy, were my thoughts as she grew smaller and smaller. I could not move until she was right out of sight.

Oh, if no one was about, it would have been so easy to have let go, and wept outright. When everyone was so happy and going home, and no more cruelly battered and mutilated bodies to help to repair. No more long hours, of praying to ask God to please spare a young man's life, so that he could at least get home, why should I feel so sad and empty. I was still young and had not suffered anything like so many had done, I now had the chance to follow my ambition, and a host of addresses from patients and colleagues alike making me feel it was not really goodbye. I hoped when I had finished my studies I would have a chance to accept their invitations and visit them all

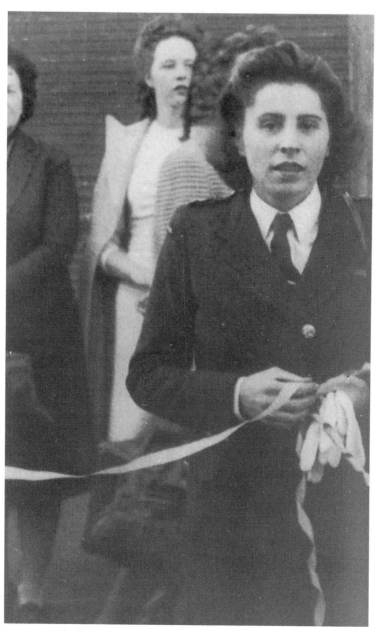

I did not move until she was right out of sight

again one day. Like the nurse at Middlesex who impressed me so much, I would not have changed my wartime occupation for any other section of it, with all it's sadness, heartaches and tears.

I could not go back to the hospital or our V.A.D.s cabins, that was once so alive with happy ever-busy V.A.D.s. Instead I made my way slowly to our club. It was a blessing one of my friends was still there, serving tea to the few remaining Kiwis still in Sydney. "Are you on your way back to the hospital, Mona?" she asked.

"I should be, but I don't want to go, it's too empty now," I quietly replied.

"Would you like to spend the night with me?" she sincerely asked.

"I'd love to," I returned and thanked her. Like a lonely lost sheep I went home with her, and was very glad I did. Over a liqueur, she told me how she had married during the last war, and had lost her infant a month before it was due, and then lost her husband who was away on active service. The world too had been very empty for her, and she had never remarried.

"We always looked forward to your coming to the club Mona," made me feel very humble. "While you have been in Sydney I have come to look upon you as my Mona. When do you think you'll get home?" That I was not going home seemed to surprise her.

"I have waited so long to take up my studies again, and continue to travel. There is more scope for me here, and in that way I won't have time to think and life can be very interesting."

"You're still young Mona, and I am sure that whoever you kept in your heart, would not expect you to fret your life away. It is very lonely to live the whole of your life out alone. Once you settle down a bit, although I know it may not be quite the same, you may meet someone else and you would be wise to marry, as you will always have children to look forward to," she advised me.

For a short while I thought over what she had said and thought what a kind, understanding person you are. One who really understood, one of the very few. We talked well into the night, and I was quite happy to return to the hospital next morning.

It was quite fun to look forward to soft boiled eggs, and not the hard boiled ones that you could play tennis with. Passing through the now almost empty grounds of the hospital it became even emptier when I reached my cabin, and saw my room-mate's empty bed. I did not even have my kitten now, as we had been told he was a she, and I had spent quite a lot of time finding a suitable home for it. I smiled to myself when I thought of Peggy, who'd had such a narrow escape with her fractured spine. Her parting words to me before she left to go on sick-leave were, "I'll drop you a line as soon as I get home Kiwi." How I laughed when her card arrived, "Hello, Menace, having a wonderful time, if you're taking temps, the answer's NO! Back to pester you soon. Love Peg."

Settling in bed that night to catch up on some of the sleep I had missed the night before, I suddenly woke with an uncanny premonition, that something was wrong. Within seconds I was wide awake, and there standing inside my cabin door was a sailor. "Get out of my room." I told him.

"I've come to talk to you," he said as he advanced towards my bed.

"Get out of my room!" I yelled at him. He disappeared. Getting straight out of bed I walked briskly along the ramps to the rec. room, and rang the guards.

"O.K. Kiwi, we're coming right over!" came across the line. As I replaced the receiver, I knew fear as I had never experienced it before. My whole body trembled. When I returned to my cabin, I rolled up my blankets, together with my mattress, and stepped across the small corridor to the cabin that faced mine, and dumped my bedding on the floor. As poor Louie sat rubbing her eyes, "It's O.K. Louie, I've had a sailor in my cabin, and I am too scared to stay alone, so I'm staying here for the rest of the night." With mild idioms they turned over and went off to sleep again.

I was struck with blank amazement, when on reporting it next morning, I was asked if I got his name and number. It went round the V.A.D. quarters like wildfire, and it soon came to light, that quite a number of the V.A.D.s had been disturbed in the night by someone in their cabins, but he disappeared as soon as he was spoken to. A couple of nights later a sailor was caught and arrested hiding under our V.A.D. quarters.

It seemed no time at all, when for the last time I would collect my Navy pay, hand in my paybook, and then commence my studies to build for myself a new and interesting way of life.

Not long after I had settled down and commenced studying, I was to receive the greatest thrill I had had for a very long time, when Bebe-De-Roland arrived in Sydney as Principal Ballerina in the show *Follow the Girls'*. No-one can imagine the thrill it was to meet her again, under such different circumstances, and have the pleasure of taking her to meet and have afternoon tea with so many of my New Zealand friends, who were her own countrymen too.

Though she was extremely busy, to watch her dance again in a different role was very stimulating, and we had time to be able to do a little sightseeing before she left to return to London.

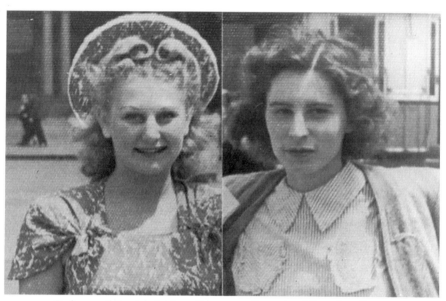

Bebe and I caught by photographers in Circular Quay,
Sydney

EPILOGUE

Every person has a life story all their own, but no life is complete unless one can be of service to others.

My V.A.D. life basically began purely on impulse, as if I had given careful thought and consideration to a way of life I knew nothing of, or to the sufferings of the sick and wounded I would have to witness and nurse, I know it would all have been lost to my typewriter.

The years I have written about, were the most colourful and gratifying I have ever found.

Though many years and an era lie between them and now, each Anzac Day carries with it, a renewal and thankfulness to all who served. Of the memories of hands of lasting friendships.

Hours of boredom, fear, action. Endless long hours given so unselfishly by so many, who, though exhausted, carried on and on in their determination to regain for us all, a peaceful and happy way of life.

As V.A.D.s we did not see the battlefields: the watery graves, the plane wreckages, or the sinister camps some of our patients were rescued from. We were also spared the shock some of the next-of-kin received, but they, together with the veterans from the Boer War, and the First World War all played their part in our mutual cause for freedom and justice.

So much depends on a nurse in peacetime, but in wartime much more must be given, as she so often is a patient's sole link with the outside world, and their relatives so many thousands of miles away. The satisfaction and disappointments of nursing of which I was made very much aware very early in my years as a Naval Nurse, convinced me that nursing is a highly individual occupation. She may not have the shorter hours of other occupations, but she has a special vocation, which carries its own reward, in seeing people as they really are. Each patient not only represents a challenge to all nursing technique, but is an individual, who requires tactful understanding.

No matter how hard we try to forget, there are still so many who lost forever relations and loved ones. There are also many who still carry permanent physical and mental scars.

History is always being made and recorded, and on the 25th. of April every year it is my privilege to remember and look back with pride on my Four Glorious Years.

Devotion

(TO A NURSE)

SURELY, before you chose this work, you prayed

Long at some starlit window, kneeling there,

For something of that starry shine has stayed

Within your eyes, it trembles in your hair.

Yours is a silver service, tipped with flame;

Yours is a trust too sacred to betray;

You never will be faithless to a name

You call your own.   O angel of night and day,

You have pledged your word to pass the busy years

In abstinence and purity; to keep

Sacred the secrets bared through pain and tears.

You have kept your pledge, your hands bring blessed sleep;

Your faith, your high devotion never fail;

You tread these halls, a modern Nightingale.

Grace Noll Crowell.